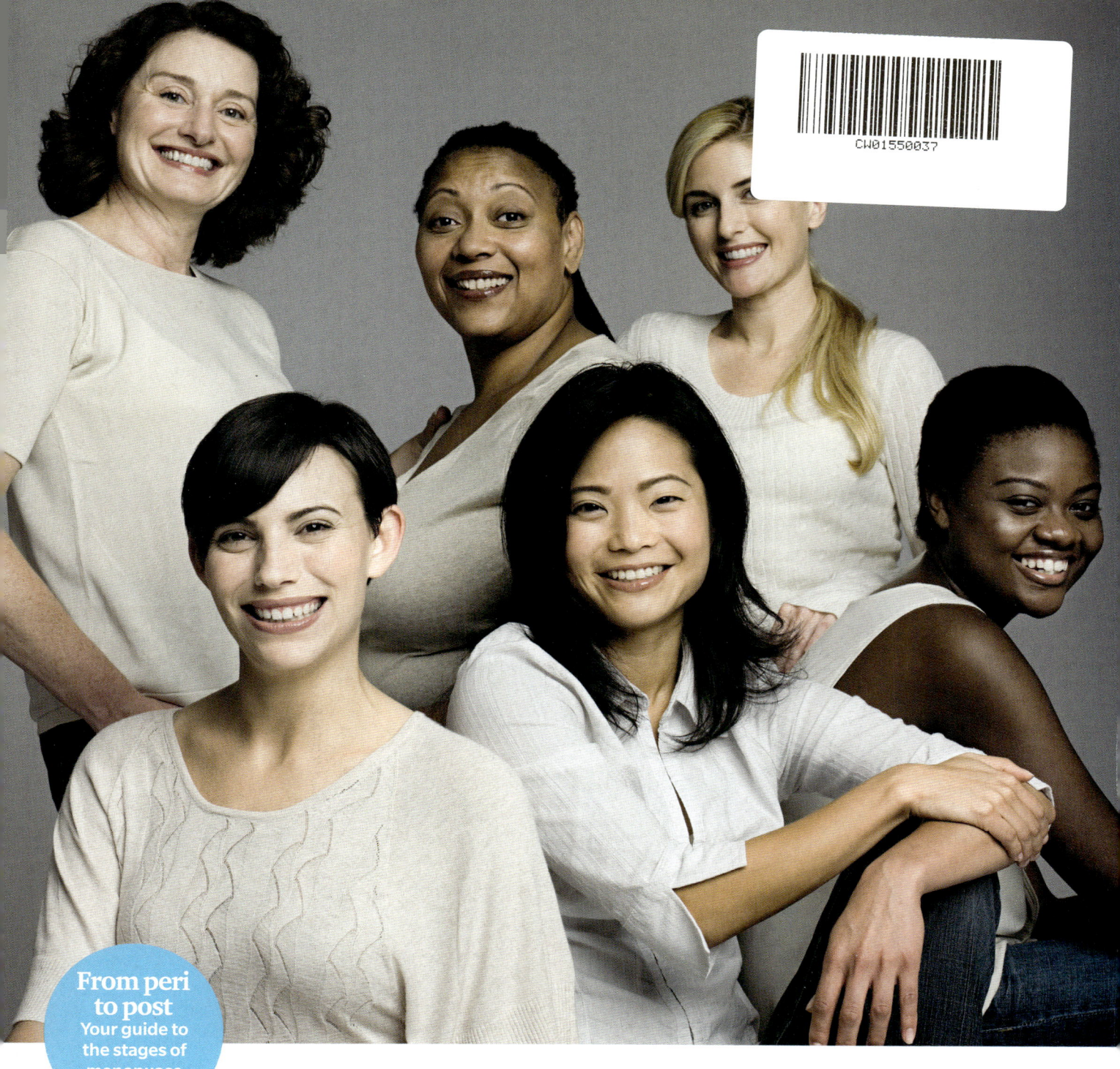

From peri to post
Your guide to the stages of menopuase starts p8.

First things first...

There's no such thing as a typical menopause. We're all different, and we'll all go through the years of 45 to 55 or so with varying degrees of disruption. But, if you've bought this bookazine, chances are you're struggling.

Perhaps you've just entered the first phase – perimenopause – and you're exhausted by sleepless nights. Or you may have landed slap-bang in the middle of full-blown menopause and you wonder if an alien (with a tendency to hot flushes and brain fog) has taken over your body.

Whichever stage you're at, there's one irrefutable truth: you're not alone. There are millions of women going through the same thing right now– and, increasingly, speaking out about it.

No longer is menopause a taboo topic. Women in midlife are pushing for greater employment rights, starting to celebrate their freedom from monthly cycles, and realising there is an exciting life to be enjoyed on the other side.

But first, let us guide you through. With hundreds of tips, personal experiences and expert advice, *The Smart Woman's Guide to the Menopause* will help you navigate the symptoms and stresses of this, your ultimate rite of passage.

The Smart Woman's Guide to the Menopause

FUTURE

THE SMART WOMAN'S GUIDE TO THE MENOPAUSE

Future PLC Quay House, The Ambury, Bath, BA1 1UA

Editorial
Lifestyle Content Director **Charlotte Richards**
Associate Editor **Michelle Hather**
Art Director **Sophie Lienard**
Compiled by **Jessica Leggett & Lora Barnes**
Senior Art Editor **Andy Downes**
Head of Art & Design **Greg Whitaker**
Editorial Director **Jon White**

Cover images
Sofie Delauw

Photography
All copyrights and trademarks are recognised and respected

Advertising
Media packs are available on request
Commercial Director **Clare Dove**

International
Head of Print Licensing **Rachel Shaw**
licensing@futurenet.com
www.futurecontenthub.com

Circulation
Head of Newstrade **Tim Mathers**

Production
Head of Production **Mark Constance**
Production Project Manager **Matthew Eglinton**
Advertising Production Manager **Joanne Crosby**
Digital Editions Controller **Jason Hudson**
Production Managers **Keely Miller, Nola Cokely, Vivienne Calvert, Fran Twentyman**

Printed in the UK

Distributed by Marketforce, 5 Churchill Place, Canary Wharf, London, E14 5HU
www.marketforce.co.uk Tel: 0203 787 9001

The Smart Woman's Guide To The Menopause Fifth Edition (LBZ4951)
© 2023 Future Publishing Limited

We are committed to only using magazine paper which is derived from responsibly managed, certified forestry and chlorine-free manufacture. The paper in this bookazine was sourced and produced from sustainable managed forests, conforming to strict environmental and socioeconomic standards.

All contents © 2023 Future Publishing Limited or published under licence. All rights reserved. No part of this magazine may be used, stored, transmitted or reproduced in any way without the prior written permission of the publisher. Future Publishing Limited (company number 2008885) is registered in England and Wales. Registered office: Quay House, The Ambury, Bath BA1 1UA. All information contained in this publication is for information only and is, as far as we are aware, correct at the time of going to press. Future cannot accept any responsibility for errors or inaccuracies in such information. You are advised to contact manufacturers and retailers directly with regard to the price of products/services referred to in this publication. Apps and websites mentioned in this publication are not under our control. We are not responsible for their contents or any other changes or updates to them. This magazine is fully independent and not affiliated in any way with the companies mentioned herein.

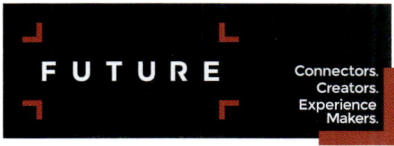

Future plc is a public company quoted on the London Stock Exchange (symbol: FUTR)
www.futureplc.com

Chief Executive **Zillah Byng-Thorne**
Non-Executive Chairman **Richard Huntingford**
Chief Financial and Strategy Officer **Penny Ladkin-Brand**

Tel +44 (0)1225 442 244

Part of the **woman** bookazine series

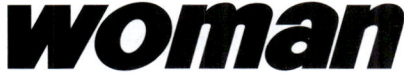

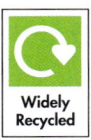
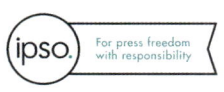

Contents

Your health

- **8** — **The three menopause stages**
  When they happen, what to expect and how to cope

- **14** — **10 things you might not know**
  We give you the lowdown and bust common myths

- **26** — **It's getting hot in here**
  There's plenty you can do to tackle those pesky flushes

- **30** — **The truth about HRT**
  Our special report will help you make an informed choice

- **36** — **Give your bones a boost**
  Strategies to reduce your risk of osteoporosis

- **44** — **Your complete guide to a stronger pelvic floor**
  Yes, you *can* overcome stress incontinence

Your looks

- **22** — **Get back to the real you**
  From weight gain to lost libido, joint pain to hair health, we're here to help

- **35** — **Her light materials**
  Dress well to keep your cool

- **40** — **Save your skin**
  Top tips for combating unwelcome changes

- **42** — **The thick of it**
  Keep your locks looking healthy and lustrous

- **72** — **Don't give in to the meno-spread**
  Make small adjustments to keep your waistline in check

- **74** — **How to ditch the menopause middle**
  21-day diet and exercise plan

Your wellbeing

- **80** — **Love and sex in midlife**
  It's different – but it can be great!

- **84** — **Talking sex**
  Your questioned answered

- **90** — **Coping with the 9 to 5**
  How to survive menopause in the workplace

- **94** — **Finding a solution…naturally**
  Non-medical remedies that work

- **98** — **CBD: your new best friend?**
  We look at the pros and cons

- **102** — **How to sleep through the menopause**
  Keep cool and drift off in comfort

- **106** — **Warning: fog ahead**
  Lift low mood and beat confusion

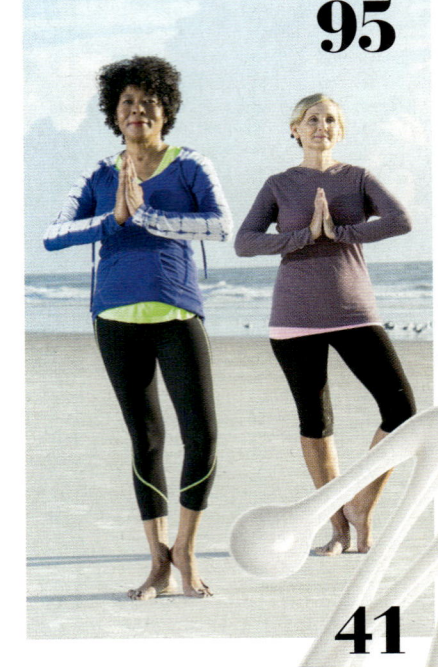
95

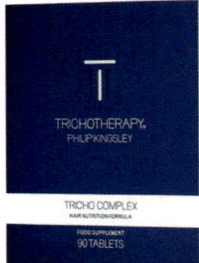
42

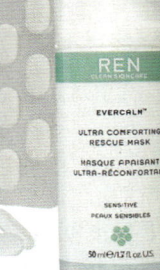
41

32

6 The Smart Woman's Guide to the Menopause

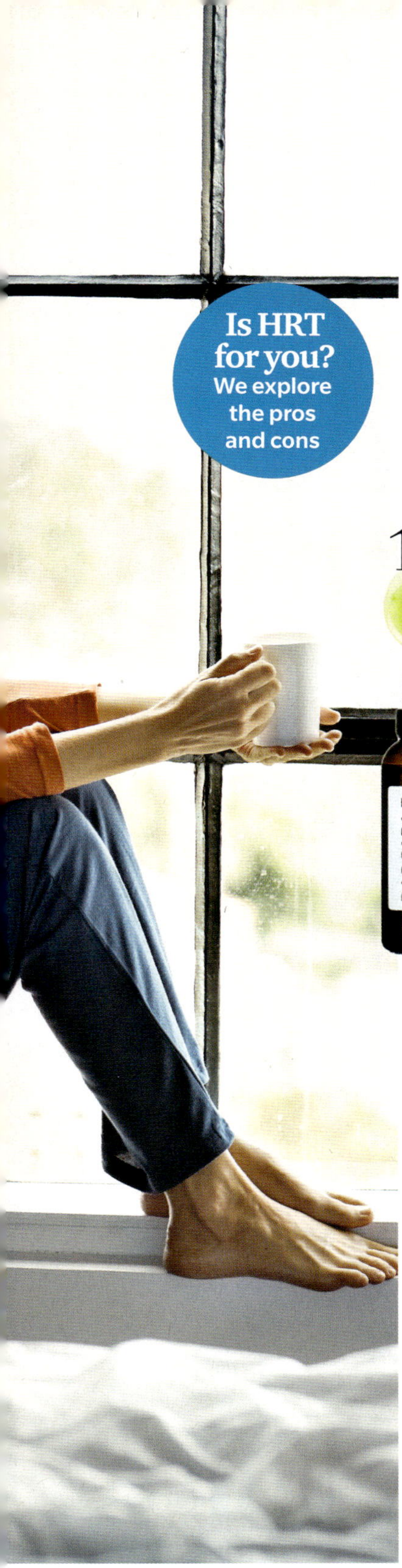

Is HRT for you? We explore the pros and cons

Diet and exercise

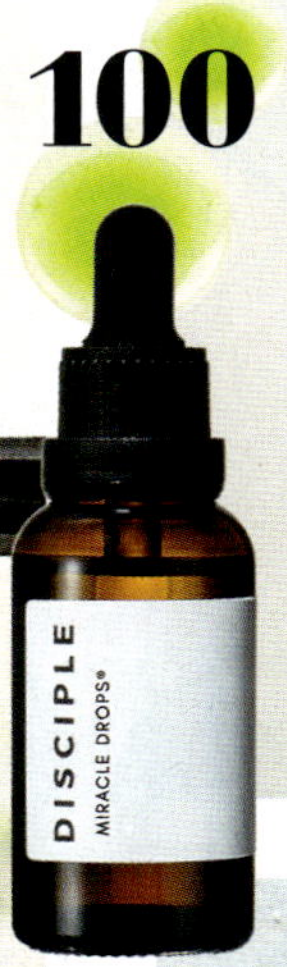

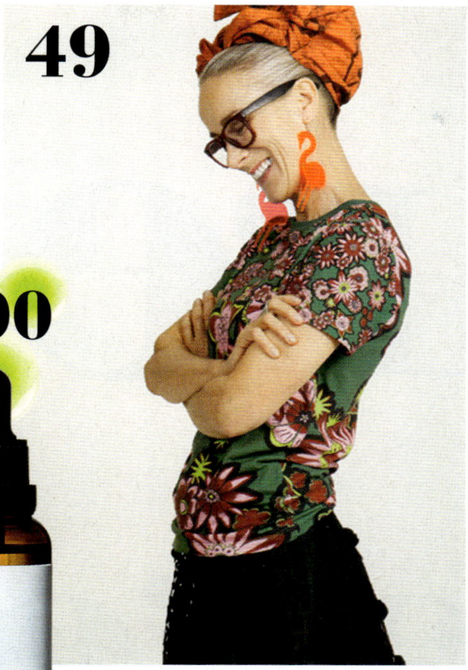

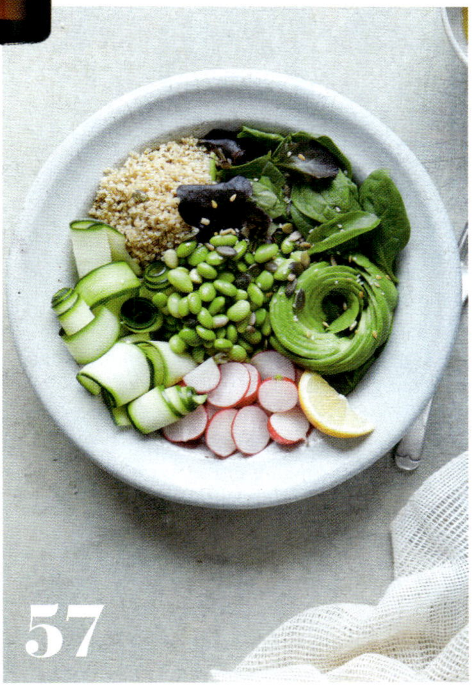

50 **Eat yourself happy and healthy**
Include these foods to enhance your mood and general wellbeing

54 **Rainbow recipes to revive you**
Tired, listless, anticipating the afternoon slump? Try these dishes

58 **Eat to beat hot flushes**
Plant-based recipes are key

62 **Feed the hormone rollercoaster**
And keep yourself on an even keel

66 **Ease your symptoms with exercise**
Get moving to boost your physical, mental and emotional wellbeing

70 **If you only do one thing…**
Walk! Set your own pace and reap the benefits, one step at a time

Inspiration

16 **Leave *no* woman behind!**
Celebs share their experiences of and thoughts on menopause

46 **The joy of change**
Journalist Caryn Franklin recounts her turbulent menopause journey

86 **Me and my menopausal vagina**
The trauma of vaginal atrophy

112 **'I thought the 90s had caught up with me…'**
Meg Mathews' insightful story

116 **5 women making a difference**
Influencers, campaigners and medics share their breakthroughs

124 **And now for the rest of your life!**
A new, exciting chapter lies ahead

128 **Be free, be brave, be happy!**
Goodbye taboos, hello liberty!

108 **Is therapy the answer?**
Some women find CBT can help

110 **The age of anxiety**
Feeling anxious is a less-known symptom of menopause

120 **The smart guide quiz**
So…how much have you learnt?

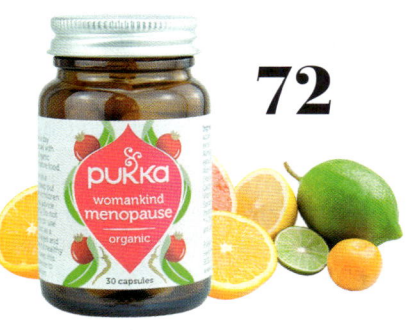

The Smart Woman's Guide to the Menopause 7

The three menopause stages

Peri, post, or just plain meno... Here's the lowdown on your stage of the 'pause'

As women, we battle against our hormones, arguably from our teenage years through to older age. And there are waves to overcome in later life, in the forms of perimenopause, menopause and postmenopause.

There was a time when 'menopause' was a forbidden word. Known as 'the change' and typified by hot flushes, mood swings, loss of libido and changes in skin, hair and body, it was nothing to celebrate, and certainly not spoken about.

Today, though, there's a different agenda. Led by women in the spotlight, from Viola Davis and Gwyneth Paltrow to Meg Mathews and Lorraine Kelly, plus a whole host of women who are writing and podcasting about the menopause, the 'M' word is becoming part of our vocabulary.

But 'menopause' is no longer a one-name-fits-all term. For every woman, it looks and feels different, and the three key stages of perimenopause, menopause and postmenopause bring their own challenges.

Whether you are at the beginning of your menopause journey, midway through or approaching the end, there's probably one thing you have in common with many other women – it's still hard to talk about. You either feel like 'the only one', or you wonder if your symptoms are the worst.

A survey from Superdrug found that 50% of women who hadn't yet experienced menopause were worried about approaching it. Symptoms that most concerned them included, at number one, hot flushes, followed by weight gain, mood swings, depression and anxiety.

Meanwhile, 63% of working women say that menopause has had a negative effect on their working life, while the British Menopause Society found that only half of women with bothersome symptoms consult their GPs for help.

Menopause has so many effects, it can be hard to know where to start to help yourself, but a good place is to understand which stage you are at or might be approaching. Read on to discover more.

Help is there
Ask your GP about easing symptoms

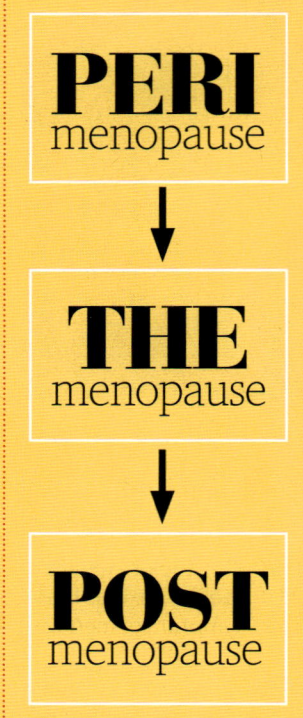

8 The Smart Woman's Guide to the Menopause

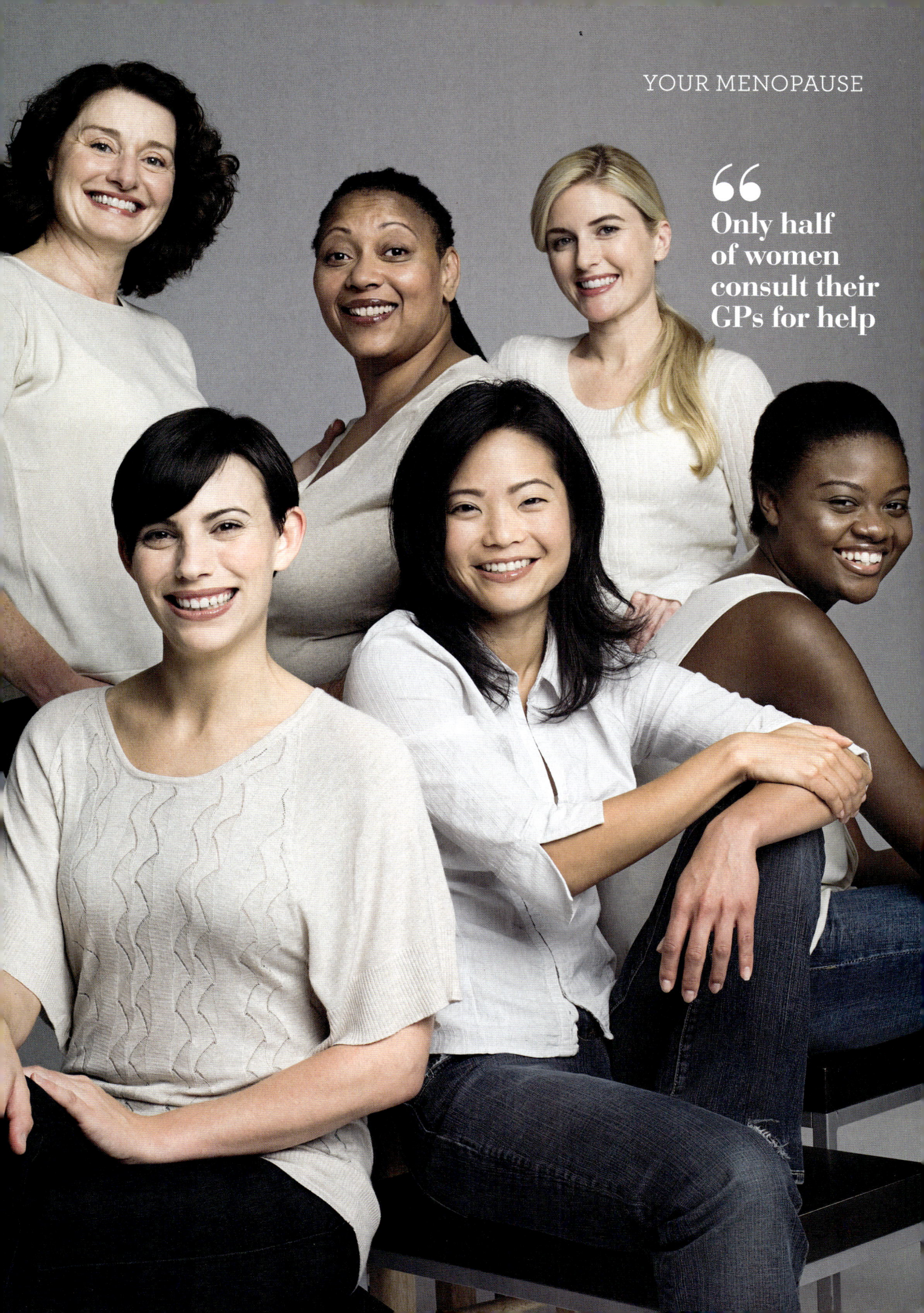

YOUR MENOPAUSE

"Only half of women consult their GPs for help

> **Menopausal symptoms can start while women are still having periods**
> *Tania Adib*

1 PERI menopause

50% of us worry about the onset of menopause

When?
Menopause typically happens between the ages of 45-55, with the average woman starting at 51.

What's happening?
Women are often unaware that they're entering the perimenopause, which can be distressing. Hot flushes and night sweats can start five or more years before your periods stop at menopause.

Dr Sarah Brewer, GP and Healthspan Medical Director, says, 'During perimenopause, ovaries produce fewer and weaker follicles until, eventually, you stop ovulating. Only 12% of women wake up one day and never have another period. The other 88% notice fluctuations, with their cycles being longer or shorter, heavier or lighter and, in some cases, with intermittent spotting.

'In early perimenopause, oestrogen levels are still high enough to allow for ovulation. However, these levels are lower than your body is used to, so symptoms may be felt before the cycle changes.'

Tania Adib, Consultant Gynaecologist at The Lister Hospital, adds, 'Menopausal symptoms can start many years before the menopause, while women are still having periods, so they often don't connect the two. Often, the levels of the hormone progesterone reduce first, causing mood swings, low mood, anxiety, poor sleep and weight gain without the classic hot flushes.

'As the ovaries "run out" of eggs, so the levels of the hormones normally produced by the ovaries reduces, and this causes symptoms of the menopause.'

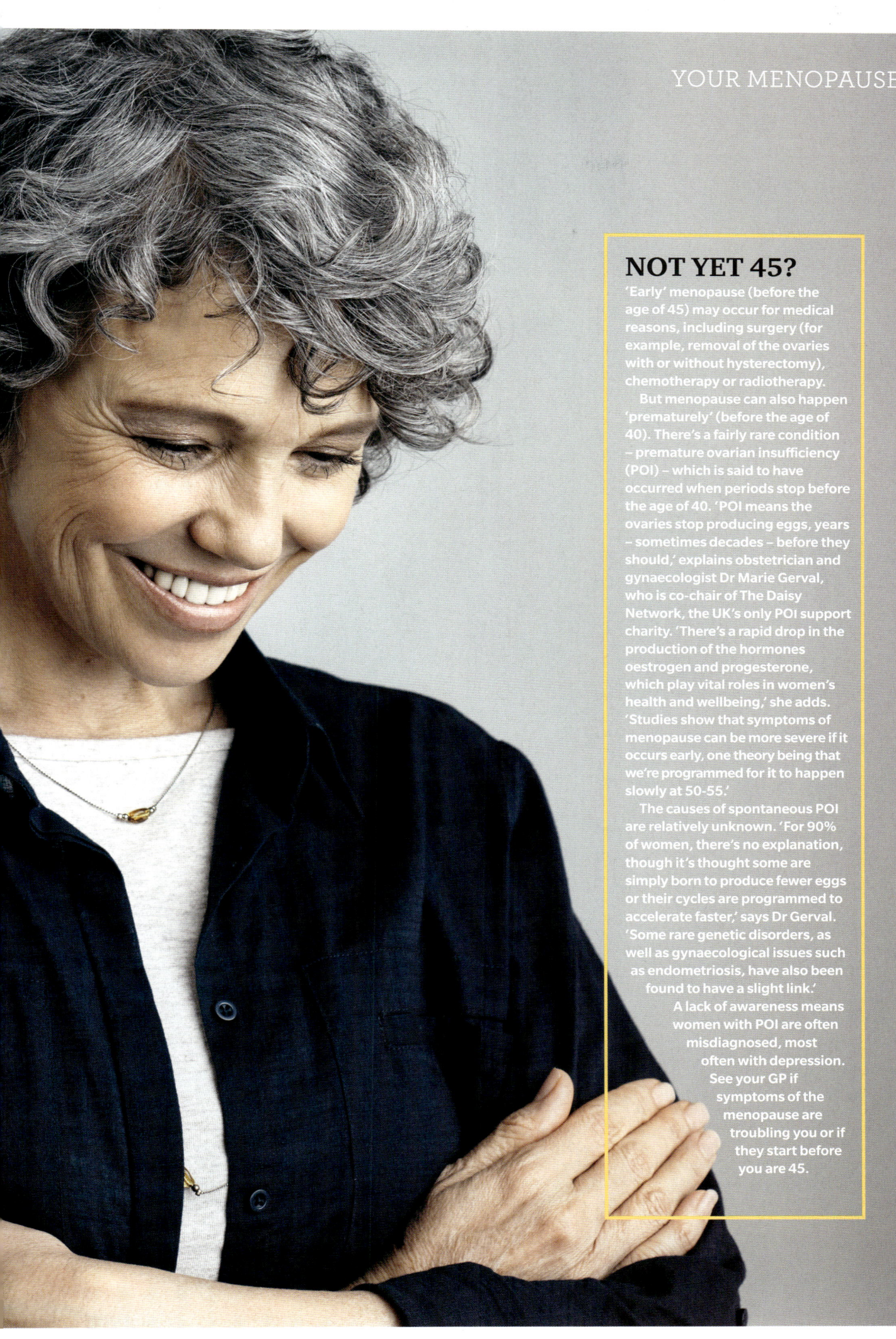

YOUR MENOPAUSE

NOT YET 45?

'Early' menopause (before the age of 45) may occur for medical reasons, including surgery (for example, removal of the ovaries with or without hysterectomy), chemotherapy or radiotherapy.

But menopause can also happen 'prematurely' (before the age of 40). There's a fairly rare condition – premature ovarian insufficiency (POI) – which is said to have occurred when periods stop before the age of 40. 'POI means the ovaries stop producing eggs, years – sometimes decades – before they should,' explains obstetrician and gynaecologist Dr Marie Gerval, who is co-chair of The Daisy Network, the UK's only POI support charity. 'There's a rapid drop in the production of the hormones oestrogen and progesterone, which play vital roles in women's health and wellbeing,' she adds. 'Studies show that symptoms of menopause can be more severe if it occurs early, one theory being that we're programmed for it to happen slowly at 50-55.'

The causes of spontaneous POI are relatively unknown. 'For 90% of women, there's no explanation, though it's thought some are simply born to produce fewer eggs or their cycles are programmed to accelerate faster,' says Dr Gerval. 'Some rare genetic disorders, as well as gynaecological issues such as endometriosis, have also been found to have a slight link.'

A lack of awareness means women with POI are often misdiagnosed, most often with depression. See your GP if symptoms of the menopause are troubling you or if they start before you are 45.

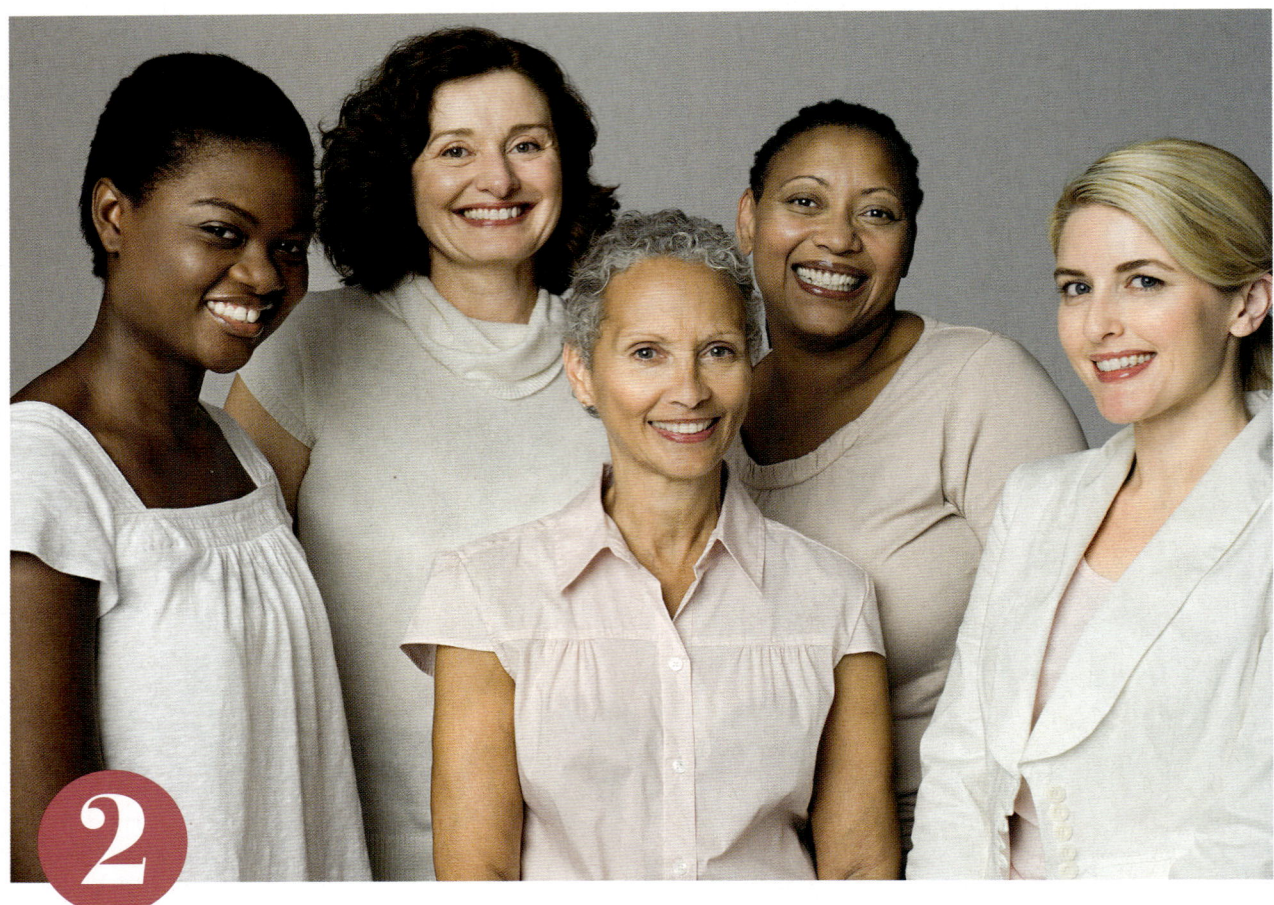

② THE menopause

> ❝ **Joints can be affected, particularly hips, knees, hands and fingers**
> *Dr Sarah Brewer*

The menopause itself is said to have been reached when a woman has been period-free for 12 continuous months.

When?
Typically, between the ages of 51-55.

What's happening?
Periods are officially over. Your ovaries no longer have enough follicles to maintain your menstrual cycle. Dr Sarah Brewer explains that, due to lack of oestrogen, joints can be affected, particularly hips and knees, as well as hands and fingers: 'Muscles, tendons and ligaments may all become more prone to stiffening and aches.'

Tania Adib says, 'The average age of the menopause is 51 in the UK, but it can start many years before that. It's estimated that around 1 in 100 women go through it under the age of 40, and 1 in 1,000 under the age of 30. When a woman has not had a period for a year, she is considered fully menopausal. However, symptoms can continue for many years after – in some cases for 10 years or more.'

She adds that as hormones (oestrogen, progesterone, testosterone and DHEA) deplete, some hormone is still produced by the adrenal glands, but very little from the ovaries. This decreased level of hormone production causes significant changes in the body.

'Some women sail through with no problems,' she says. 'Others have terrible symptoms which very significantly affect the quality of their lives and can cause loss of confidence and problems coping at work and socially. Even if they have no symptoms, over time they will be more at risk of heart disease and osteoporosis. They may also experience vaginal dryness, the need to go to the toilet to pass urine more frequently, incontinence and prolapse.'

While the symptoms listed as part of perimenopause are also part and parcel of the menopause, there is plenty we can do, from recognising them to seeking natural solutions, diet, exercise and even therapy.

YOUR MENOPAUSE

3
POST
menopause

What's happening?
After the menopause, the adrenal glands continue producing small amounts of a type of oestrogen called oestrone. Excess stress can reduce this adrenal output, so de-stressing is key.

Dr Brewer explains, 'Progesterone levels fall to as little as one-twentieth of premenopausal levels, which may contribute to some postmenopausal symptoms, such as mood swings.'

Eat yourself better
Healthy fats and foods rich in vitamin C can help boost libido

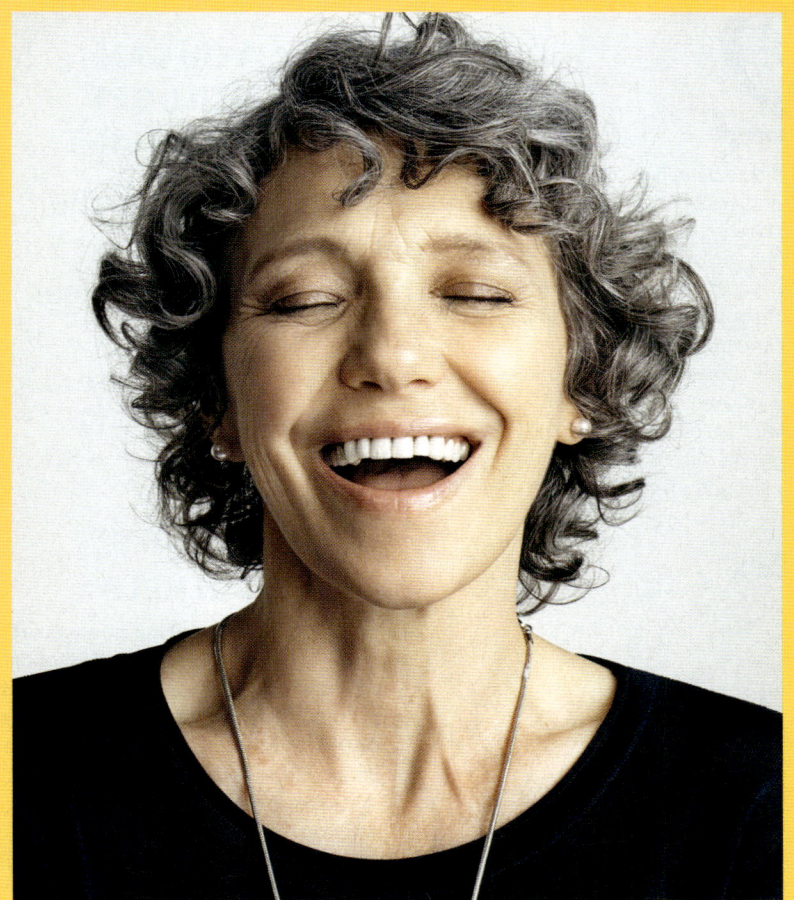

YOUR HORMONES EXPLAINED
These hormones are essential for every aspect of life, but what's what?

OESTROGEN
Nutritionist Yvonne Bishop-Weston explains that, in the thick of the menopause, ovaries stop producing as much oestrogen. 'This, along with tailed-off progesterone, can impact on bone health and be an osteoporosis risk factor. It also leads to symptoms such as thinning skin and hair, loss of skin elasticity, low mood and vaginal dryness.'

PROGESTERONE
Premenopause, progesterone is produced by the ovaries after ovulation, typically halfway through the monthly cycle. 'In perimenopause, women ovulate less often, so have the oestrogen but not the balancing progesterone,' says Yvonne. 'This period of oestrogen dominance can lead to irregular periods and mood swings.' Tania adds that progesterone can 'normalise blood clotting, reduce hot flushes, restore libido and regulate blood sugars.'

TESTOSTERONE
Primarily a male sex hormone, this is produced by women, too. 'In women, testosterone increases libido, boosts muscle mass and strength, increases energy levels and improves mood, vitality, memory and bone density,' says Tania, adding that low levels can cause fatigue, irritability, depression, and decreased bone density. It's also vital in preventing heart disease.

OXYTOCIN
AKA 'the love drug', Alison Cullen, nutritionist for A.Vogel, explains that oxytocin can fall during menopause, causing a drop in libido. Magnesium and cholesterol are needed for its formation, as is vitamin C. Eating healthy fats like avocados, walnuts and olives help keep 'good' cholesterol levels up, while vitamin C is present in all fresh fruit and veg.

The Smart Woman's Guide to the Menopause

10 things you **might not know** about the MENOPAUSE

Whether you have endless symptoms or sail through, we're here to inject a little clarity into the chaos

1 IT'S NOT ALL BAD
You might feel more creative, more balanced, more liberated. Without monthly periods and PMS, women often feel more capable, empowered – and *do* find joy in life.

2 'End of monthly cycles'
That's the definition of the word 'menopause', and it means you're only considered to have reached it when you've had no periods for a year. Before this – during perimenopause – your periods may become more erratic, longer, shorter or lighter. Studies show the median length from perimenopause to finish is 7.5 years – roughly three before your last period and 4.5 after.

3 Not everyone suffers from hot flushes
A lucky 25% of women never get them, but if you're in the unlucky 75%, avoid what makes them worse, like alcohol, spicy foods and smoking. Wear cotton sleepwear and have a fan by your bed. Regular exercise helps, too.

4 YOU CAN STILL GET PREGNANT
Don't throw away the contraceptives just yet! You need to wait until a year after your last period – or two years if you're under 50.

5 HERBALS CAN HELP
'Research has shown that black cohosh and St John's wort are effective in relieving symptoms, particularly when taken together,' says Dr Dick Middleton, former chair of the British Herbal Medicine Association. 'Anti-stress herbs valerian and Avena sativa are great for adrenal support, and sage helps with hot flushes,' says nutritional therapist Alison Cullen.

NEED-TO-KNOW

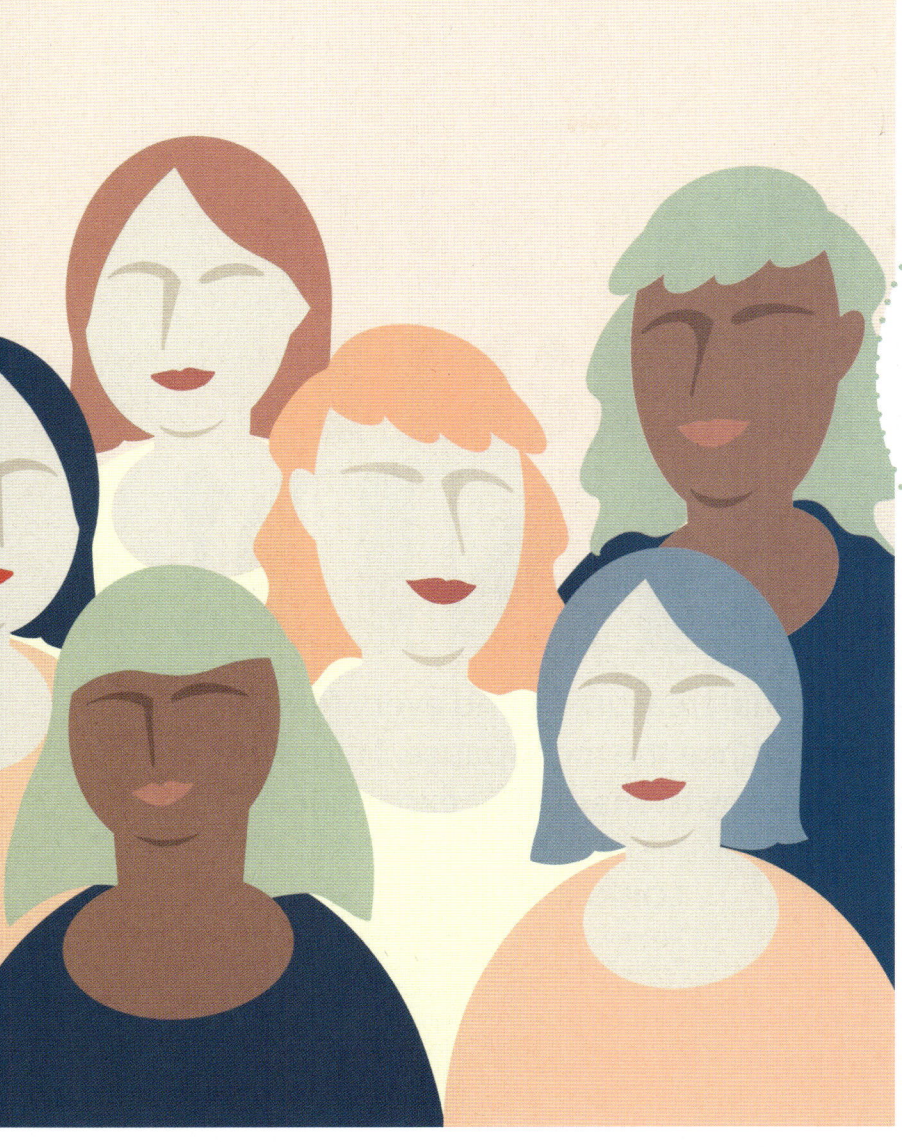

8 MOVING AROUND CAN RELIEVE MOODS

The menopause often coincides with other life stresses, such as work pressures, ageing parents and children leaving home, all of which can affect your mood. Regular exercise, yoga, meditation or simply making time for yourself can all lift your mood.

9 Switch red wine for white

While all types of alcohol can cause the release of the hormone epinephrine, triggering a hot flush, red wine is especially potent. White wine is more likely to leave you flush-free – but, as all alcohol raises your risk of breast cancer, do drink moderately.

6 It's normal to be a bit leaky

(especially when you laugh or sneeze). Falling oestrogen levels can make your pelvic floor muscles weaken – but don't ever suffer in silence. Do pelvic-floor exercises religiously, and, if the problems persist, see your doctor or continence specialist. You're not alone!

7 MEMORY LOSS ISN'T PERMANENT

Regularly forget your keys or wonder why you walked into a room? This is completely normal. Scientists believe the drop in oestrogen can make us feel a bit foggy, particularly during the perimenopause. Good news is it usually only lasts a year.

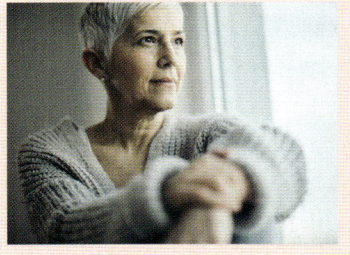

10 YOUR PURSE WILL THANK YOU

The end of periods means no more tampons or towels – and, after probably 40 years of buying them, that's quite a relief. Moneysavingexpert.com reckons a woman can spend up to £70 a year and £2,730 over the course of her lifetime on branded products. If you're still having periods, check out the website's guide to cutting the cost of sanitary protection.

The Smart Woman's Guide to the Menopause

Leave *no* woman BEHIND!

From Hollywood stars to national treasures – and every female on the planet – we will all experience the menopause. Here's our round-up of celebrities happy to share their experiences

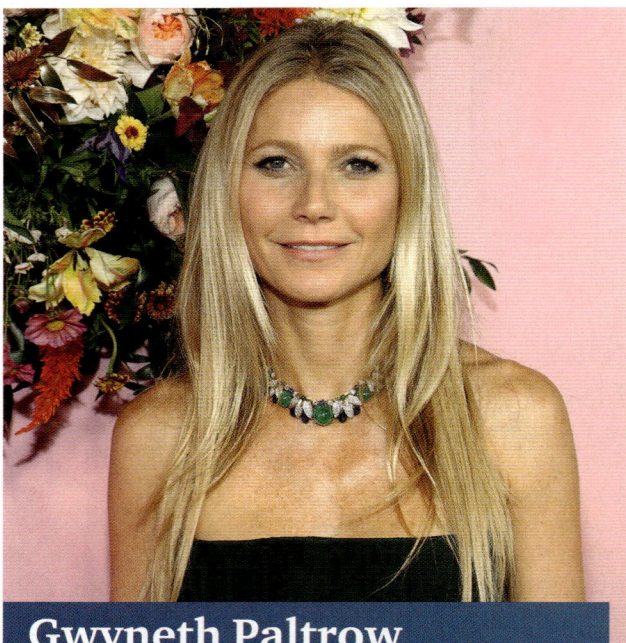

Gwyneth Paltrow
She's a cheerleader for wellbeing, although her Goop site features products that are often ridiculed – vaginal steamer, anyone? – but Gwynnie, 49, is a true champion of the menopause. After noticing perimenopausal symptoms, she has said she'd like the experience to be 'rebranded'. 'You're just all of a sudden furious for no reason,' she admitted. 'I don't think we have in our society a great example of an aspirational menopausal woman.'

LORRAINE KELLY
Queen of daytime TV Lorraine credits exercise and HRT with easing her symptoms, saying, 'We were talking last year about menopause and how difficult it can be for everybody. Sometimes I feel completely overwhelmed. I'm better now I've got HRT, and I swear by it. I know it's not for everybody. I did get quite anxious, and [exercise] really helps with that.'

Lorraine, 62, often posts sweaty selfies on Instagram after Zumba classes, and her renewed love of fitness has impacted her mental wellbeing. She told Dr Hilary Jones, 'Like so many people, I found excuses not to commit to a regular exercise routine. But, after finding exercise I really enjoy, and going to classes regularly, I feel better, not only physically but also mentally.'

> *I feel better, not only physically, but also mentally*
> **Lorraine Kelly**

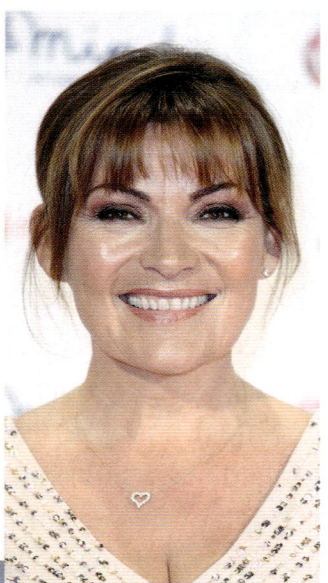

16 The Smart Woman's Guide to the Menopause

EXPERIENCE

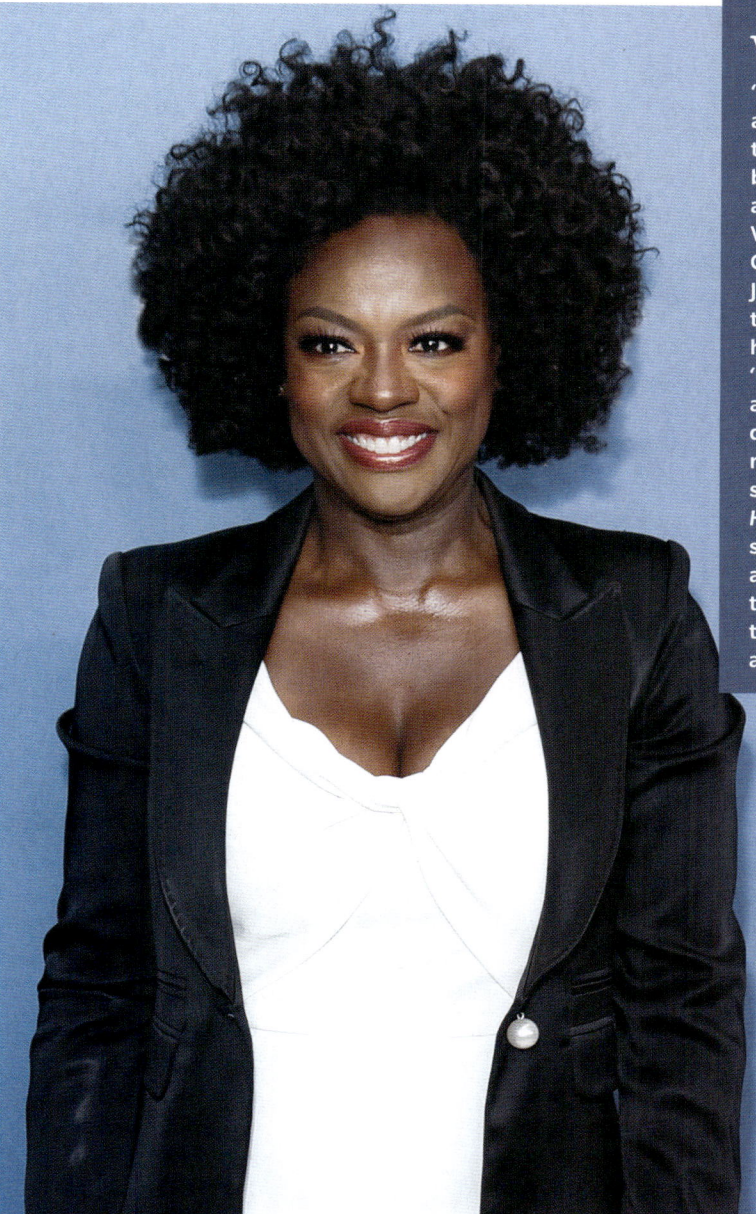

Viola Davis

'Hell' and a 'dark hole' are disturbing terms to describe menopause, but that's what multi-award-winning actress Viola Davis, 56, has said. Chatting to talk-show host Jimmy Kimmel, she added that she could love or hate her husband all in one day. 'When you talk about anything, especially dealing with menopause… men just die a slow death,' said the star of *Widows*, *The Help* and *Fences*, for which she won a best supporting actress Oscar. She added that she had been going through symptoms for around 'six to seven years'.

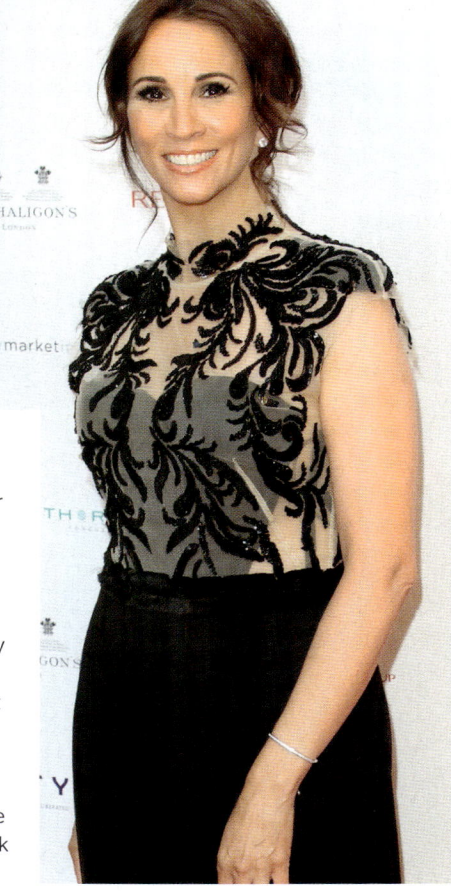

ANDREA MCLEAN

The *Loose Women* presenter feels so passionately about the menopause, she wrote a book, *Confessions of a Menopausal Woman,* and has spoken frankly over the years about the challenges – and intimacy. She's said women should be able to wear 'Menopause on Board' badges so they get space or a seat on public transport. 'At some point, we're all going to go through the menopause, and the more open I am about it, the better,' said Andrea, 52.

Sex is different
Andrea said our bodies and minds are inextricably linked.

'Whatever your experience of sex has been throughout your life – good, bad or indifferent – the menopause is one of those times when it most definitely changes. If, like me, you've had children, then it's right up there with post-baby sex – you either get right back in the saddle or you grit your teeth and bear it while internally raging that this is yet another thing you have to do.

'[A woman's body] changes during the menopause – it just doesn't seem to work the way it used to.'

The Smart Woman's Guide to the Menopause

Gillian Anderson

Star of *The X-Files* and *The Fall*, the actress, now 53, has shared how overwhelmed she felt in perimenopause. 'It was at the point that I felt like my life was falling apart around me that I started to ask what could be going on internally, and friends suggested it might be hormonal…

'I was used to being able to balance a lot of things, and all of a sudden I felt like I could handle nothing. I felt completely overwhelmed,' she said. 'Perimenopause and menopause should be treated as the rites of passage that they are – and, if not celebrated, then at least accepted and acknowledged and honoured.'

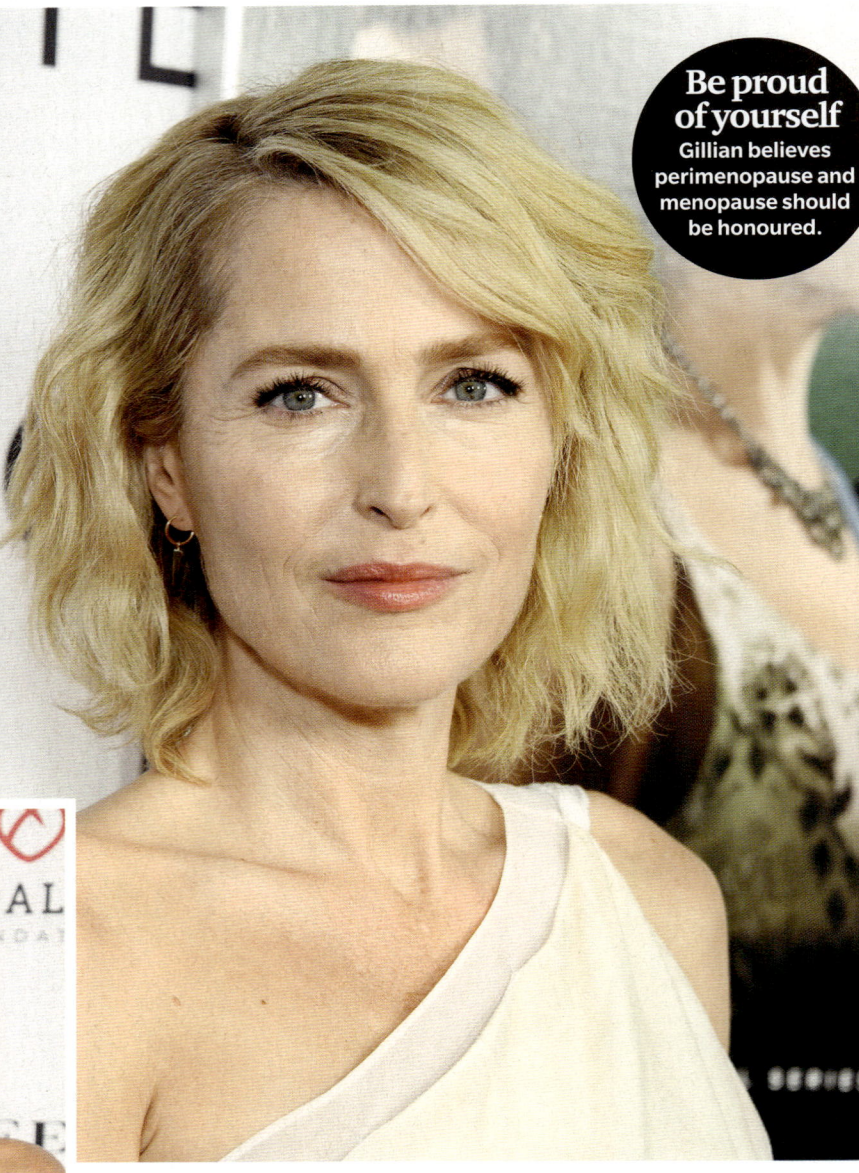

Be proud of yourself
Gillian believes perimenopause and menopause should be honoured.

DENISE VAN OUTEN

Revealing that she thought she was going 'crazy' before she was finally diagnosed with perimenopause (a diagnosis that then made her cry with relief) the 47-year-old former presenter of *The Big Breakfast* and former *Loose Women* regular admitted during an appearance on *Lorraine*: 'I didn't know straightaway. I went to get checked because my GP had said to me "I think you should go for a hormone test". And then everything just made sense.

'When I got the results, I sat there and I cried, and I thought, "I'm not going crazy!"

'It came out of the blue for me because I'm perimenopausal, and it was something that obviously now we all talk about – and I think it's brilliant! – but it was never talked about before.'

Denise stressed the importance of menopause being more widely discussed and publicised so that women are more aware and don't feel isolated. 'I've experienced hormonal-related anxiety and depression recently, and it's a horrible place to be. Don't suffer in silence,' she advises.

EXPERIENCE

AMANDA REDMAN

The 64-year-old actress, who has starred in such popular TV series as *New Tricks* and *The Good Karma Hospital,* told *The Telegraph* newspaper she felt sorry for older women who had gone through the menopause when it was more of a taboo.

'How hideous for women of our mothers' generation, because – while me and my girlfriends will talk about everything under the sun, including the menopause – it was something they didn't discuss. They must have felt so lonely and embarrassed all the time.'

Amanda admits that, although the worst is over, she's not yet symptom-free: 'For me, it's tailing off now. But I can still suddenly go that awful colour when I'm talking to somebody, and sweat beads will break out on my upper lip. You're acutely aware of it, even if they're not. The more open we are about it, the less of a taboo it will become.'

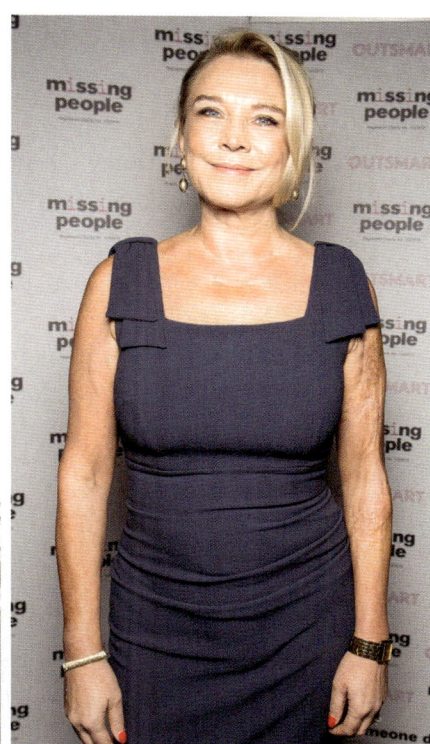

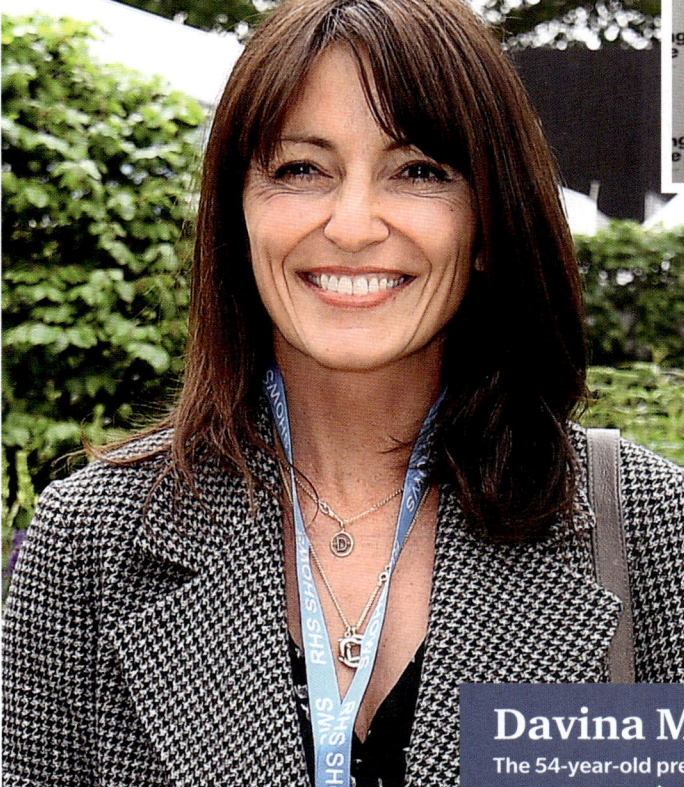

> Once you've got your head around that change, the next phase is really exciting
> *Davina McCall*

Davina McCall

The 54-year-old presenter is happy to share her experience of menopause, saying, 'People think it's something that happens in your 50s, but it didn't for me. I got the perimenopause at 44. I felt embarrassed and like I was really unattractive. I also felt unfeminine and old. Actually, I'm here to say that you can get through it.' Davina chose to go on HRT, but says it's important for every woman to do her research and find the help that is right for her. 'The menopause is not the end of your life – it's a time of change,' she says. 'Once you've got your head around that change, the next phase of your life is really exciting. You start realising, "Now I can start thinking about where I want to be in the next period of my life"'.

The Smart Woman's Guide to the Menopause

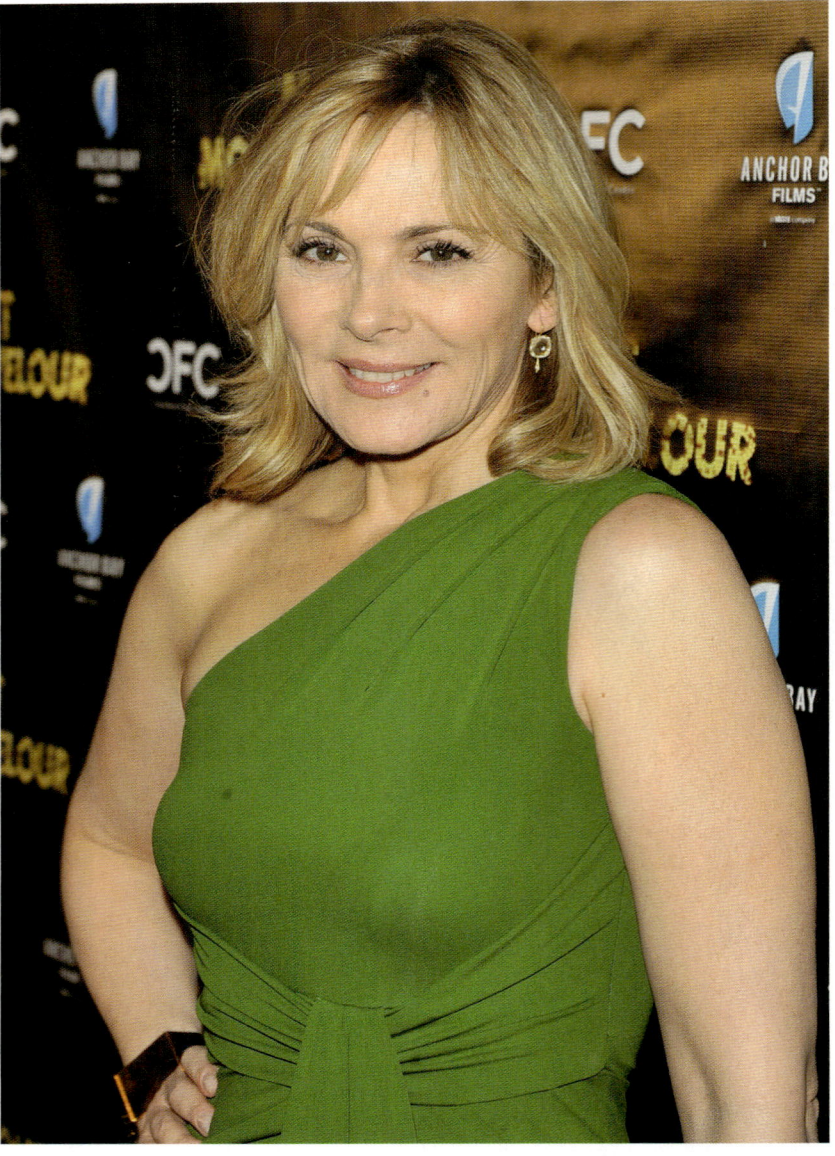

Change is part of being human. We evolve and should not fear that change
Kim Cattrall

KIM CATTRALL

The British-Canadian actress portrayed the menopause memorably in her role in *Sex and the City*, playing Samantha Jones, and Kim, now 65, has been open about her own experiences. 'Literally one moment you're fine, and then another, you feel like you're in a vat of boiling water, and you feel like the rug has been pulled out from underneath you — especially the first experience,' she has said. 'But change is part of being human. We evolve and should not fear that change.

'You're not alone. I feel that part of living this long is experiencing this, so I'm trying to turn it into a very positive thing for myself – which it has been, in the sense of acceptance and tolerance and education about this time of life.'

YOUR ROAD TO FREEDOM

Phoebe Waller-Bridge, 36, is years off the menopause, but she wrote a great speech for her acclaimed series *Fleabag*, delivered by fellow actor Kristin Scott Thomas, about what it is to be a woman. If you're struggling, read it to yourself daily:

'Women are born with pain built in. It's our physical destiny: period pains, sore boobs, childbirth… We carry it within ourselves throughout our lives…

'We have it all going on in here inside, we have pain on a cycle for years and years and years – and then, just when you feel you are making peace with it all, what happens? The menopause comes, the f***ing menopause comes, and it is the most wonderful f***ing thing in the world. And yes, your entire pelvic floor crumbles and you get f***ing hot and no-one cares, but then you're free, no longer a slave, no longer a machine with parts. You're just a person.' We hear you, Phoebe!

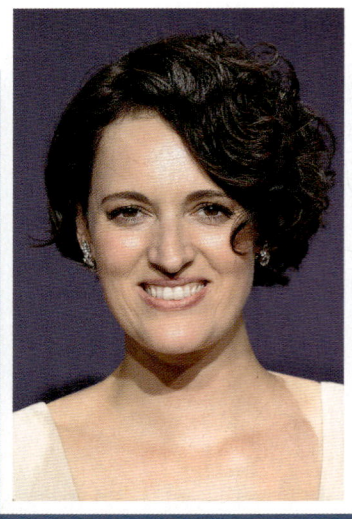

EXPERIENCE

Carol Vorderman

After finding fame on *Countdown*, Carol, 60, has survived the *I'm a Celebrity* jungle, but menopause left her feeling depressed. 'I'd wake up and think, "I don't see the point in carrying on, I just don't see the point in life", and there was no reason to feel that way,' she explained. 'I went through this terrible hormonal depression – and I don't use that word lightly. It really was awful.' She credits some special bioidentical gels with helping her through, and that trusty friend exercise – Carol does squats and goes hiking in the Brecon Beacons.

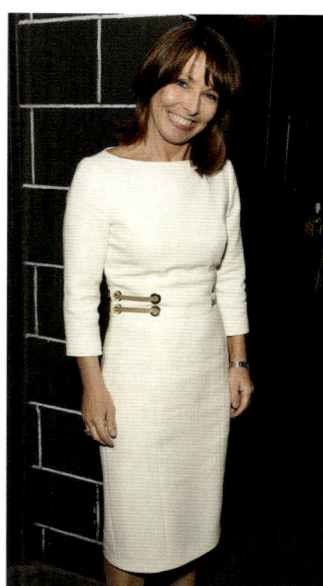

KAY BURLEY

She might seem super-confident when she's presenting *Sky News* on weekdays but, for Kay Burley, 60, the hot sweats of menopause mean regular make-up touch-ups during ad breaks, and she has discussed how she takes a herbal remedy to help with symptoms. She told mpoweredwomen.net: 'I felt I needed to broach the subject of the menopause with some of the young boys at the office, as they'd be thinking, "Why is she so hot and bothered?" Sweat would literally be dripping off my top lip and they didn't know where to look. I described it as a "power surge", and now I say, "Just having a power surge, nothing to worry about. It'll be gone in a minute".'

The Smart Woman's Guide to the Menopause

Take steps today
There are many ways you can make a difference

Get back to the real you

When everything in life appears to be changing out of your control, here's how to feel like you again…

For many years, the menopause was known as 'the change' – and not without reason. From your waistline to your mood, joint pain to complexion, the symptoms can transform your body and make you feel older than your years. 'It's a time of transition,' says pelvic floor specialist Jane Wake (janewake.com). 'It's a huge hormonal shift that affects both the physical and mental aspects of a woman's life.'

But you can reverse the changes menopause brings, and even use some of them to your advantage. Here's how…

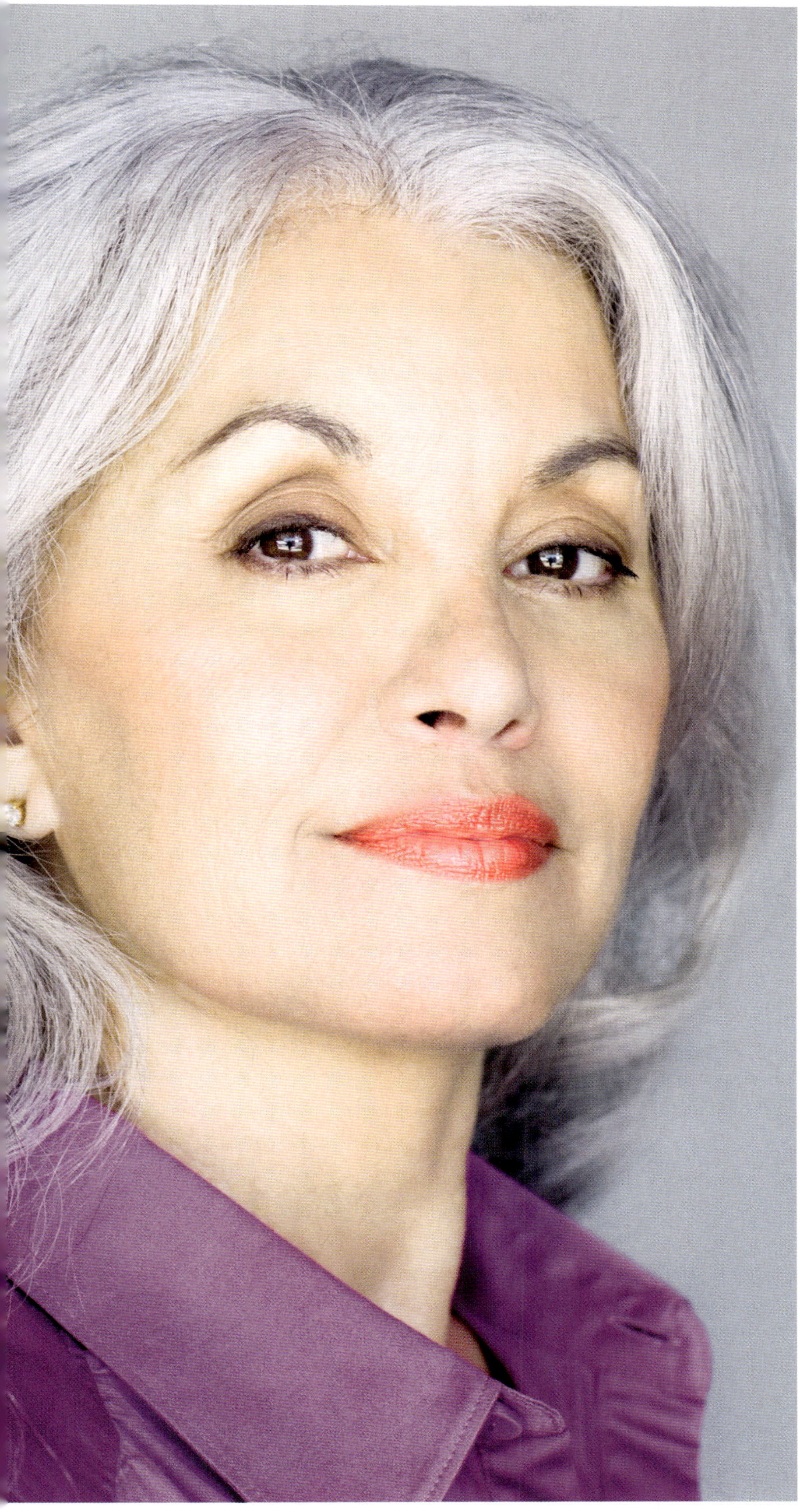

TAKE BACK CONTROL

It's a time of transition, physically and mentally
Jane Wake

Reboot your bones
During and postmenopause, women lose essential bone mass or density. 'One in three menopausal women will suffer osteoporosis,' says pharmacist Dr Omar Milhem. But staying active can reverse bone decline.
TRY: Gentle press-ups against a wall to strengthen wrists; lift food tins or squeeze a tennis ball while watching TV; strengthen hips by standing on one leg for one minute three times a day.
We're here to help, p36.

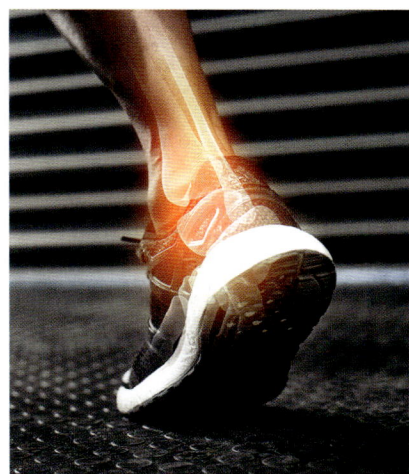

Reverse that middle-age spread
No, you're not imagining your weight gain – women entering perimenopause can put on pounds. 'The drop in oestrogen levels has the effect of redistributing body fat, so excess pounds settle around the waist,' says consultant gynaecologist Tania Adib. Don't aim for the shape you

The Smart Woman's Guide to the Menopause

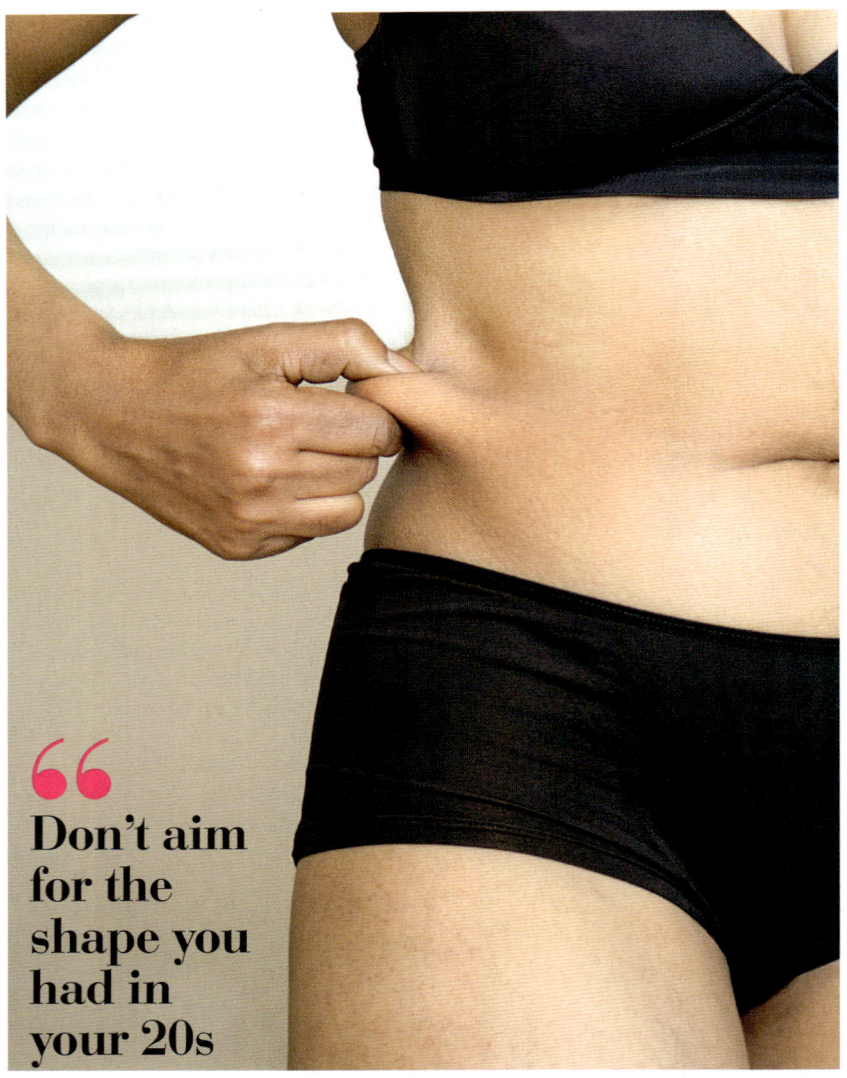

> Don't aim for the shape you had in your 20s

Ease joint pain
'Menopausal joint pain can start years before other symptoms,' says consultant rheumatologist Dr Rod Hughes. 'This is due to declining oestrogen levels, causing a reduction in collagen, loss of cartilage and an increase in inflammation.' Consider taking a supplement, such as **LithoLexal Marine Plant Extract (£24.95 for one month's supply of 60 capsules, holland andbarrett.com)**.

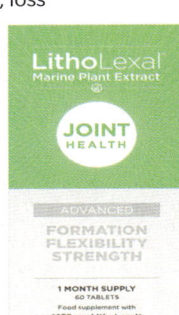

Reclaim your crown
Just over a third of women with thinning hair aged 45-59 identify the menopause as a trigger. Your hair may not grow as long before falling out, either. Low iron can be the reason. 'Eat plenty of leafy, green veg, beetroot, pistachios, blackcurrants, dried apricots, pumpkin seeds, sunflower seeds, cashews, lentils, chickpeas, prunes and kidney beans,' says nutritional therapist Alison Cullen. If there's no improvement after three months, ask your GP to check for low thyroid function.
We're here to help, p42.

had in your 20s, but a healthy weight, so your risk of arthritis, diabetes and heart disease is low. 'Cut down portion sizes and base meals around proteins, healthy fats and vegetables,' says nutritionist Rob Hobson.
We're here to help, p72.

Re-tighten your pelvic floor
'Over 50% of all women experiencing the menopause suffer from urge or stress urinary incontinence as a result,' says Jane Wake. But, if you put in the work, your pelvic floor can return to its former glory. Try Jane's easy exercise several times a day.
THE LIFT: Imagine your pelvic floor is a lift going up five floors. Pull up a little (20%), that's first floor, then a bit more to 2nd floor (40% effort), and so on until you reach the 5th floor. Then lower back down slowing, aiming to stop at each floor.
We're here to help, p44.

Stop the sag
Sadly, there is no magic cream to reduce wrinkles, but you can help reduce the signs of menopause from your skin, such as dryness, sagging and a lack of glow. 'To preserve collagen and elastin, there are key things to avoid,' says Dr Julia Sevi from Aesthetic Health. 'The biggest culprits are sunlight, smoking, pollution and stress.' Including nuts, seeds and legumes in your daily diet can help your skin regain its youthful glow.
We're here to help, p40.

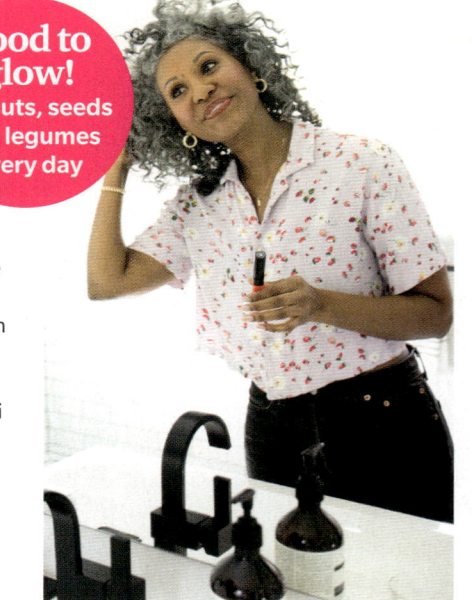

Food to glow! Eat nuts, seeds and legumes every day

TAKE BACK CONTROL

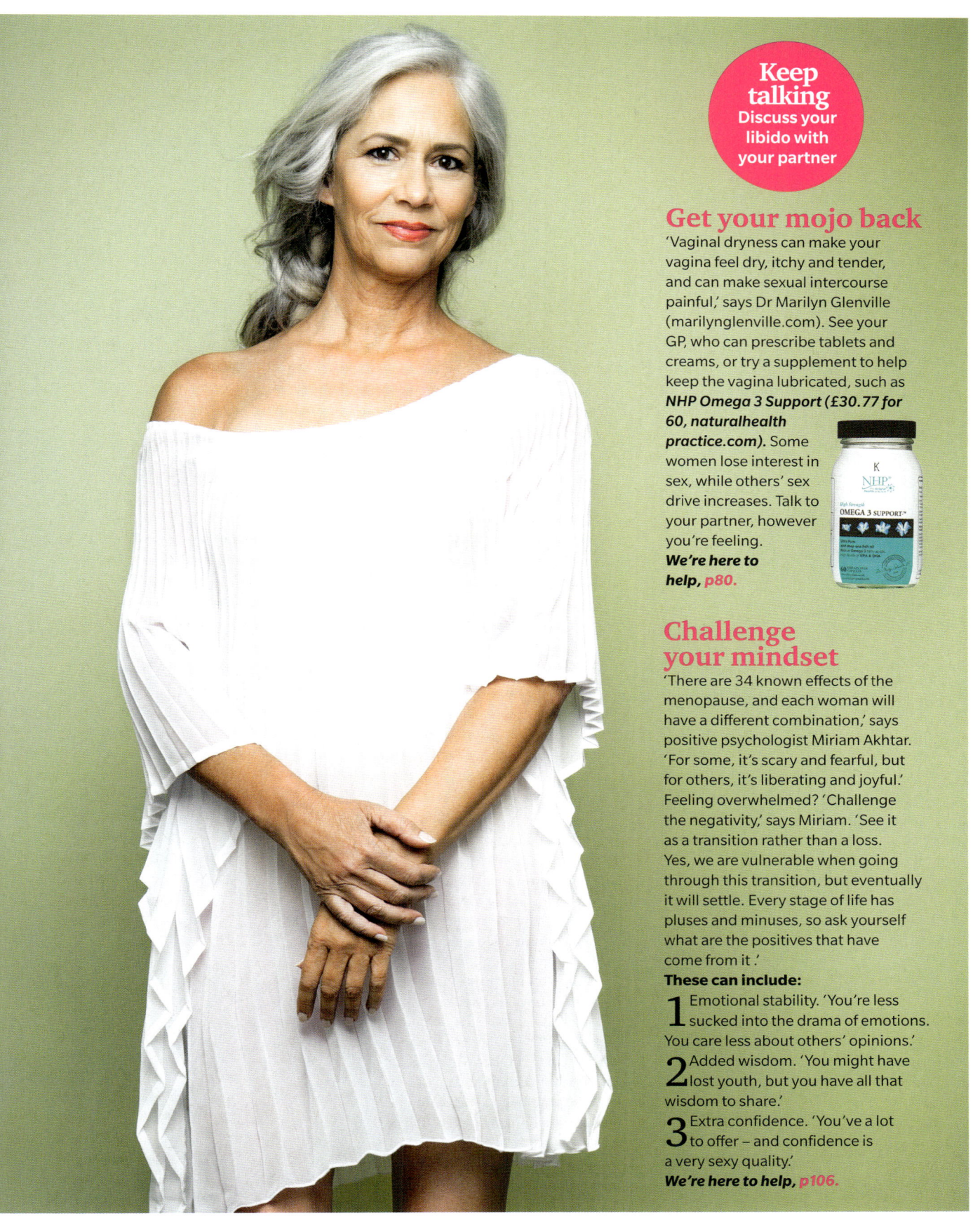

Keep talking Discuss your libido with your partner

Get your mojo back

'Vaginal dryness can make your vagina feel dry, itchy and tender, and can make sexual intercourse painful,' says Dr Marilyn Glenville (marilynglenville.com). See your GP, who can prescribe tablets and creams, or try a supplement to help keep the vagina lubricated, such as **NHP Omega 3 Support (£30.77 for 60, naturalhealth practice.com).** Some women lose interest in sex, while others' sex drive increases. Talk to your partner, however you're feeling. **We're here to help, p80.**

Challenge your mindset

'There are 34 known effects of the menopause, and each woman will have a different combination,' says positive psychologist Miriam Akhtar. 'For some, it's scary and fearful, but for others, it's liberating and joyful.' Feeling overwhelmed? 'Challenge the negativity,' says Miriam. 'See it as a transition rather than a loss. Yes, we are vulnerable when going through this transition, but eventually it will settle. Every stage of life has pluses and minuses, so ask yourself what are the positives that have come from it.'

These can include:

1. Emotional stability. 'You're less sucked into the drama of emotions. You care less about others' opinions.'
2. Added wisdom. 'You might have lost youth, but you have all that wisdom to share.'
3. Extra confidence. 'You've a lot to offer – and confidence is a very sexy quality.'

We're here to help, p106.

The Smart Woman's Guide to the Menopause 25

It's getting HOT IN HERE

The commonest and perhaps most bothersome aspect of menopause is an out-of-control body thermostat. Here's how to keep your cool...

You've dressed for the weather, done your hair and make-up when, suddenly, whoosh! Here comes an intense heat that has you stripping off layers, your hair damp, foundation sliding down your face. Around 60-80% of perimenopausal women experience hot flushes, but there are things you can do.

Are they inevitable?

Not all women get them – but, for some, they are so severe that they make life a misery. The good news is you rarely look as hot as you feel, and often the only outward sign is slight blushing – and what may feel like a soaking sweat may be barely noticeable to people around you.

What causes flushes?

Experts are unsure, but latest thinking is that it's due to several factors. 'Flushes occur when the "thermoneutral zone" – the band of temperature at which you feel comfortable – shrinks,' explains David Sturdee, President of the International Menopause Society and a spokesman for the Royal College of Obstetricians and Gynaecologists. 'It's thought oestrogen "primes" the body to react to temperature change, and that fluctuating levels at menopause cause the body to become sensitive to the slightest rise.' In addition, it's thought that over-activity of stress hormone noradrenaline and lower levels of serotonin may also be involved.

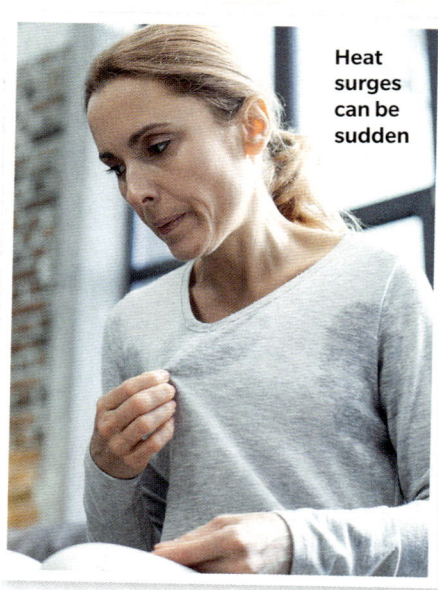

Heat surges can be sudden

BODY THERMOSTAT

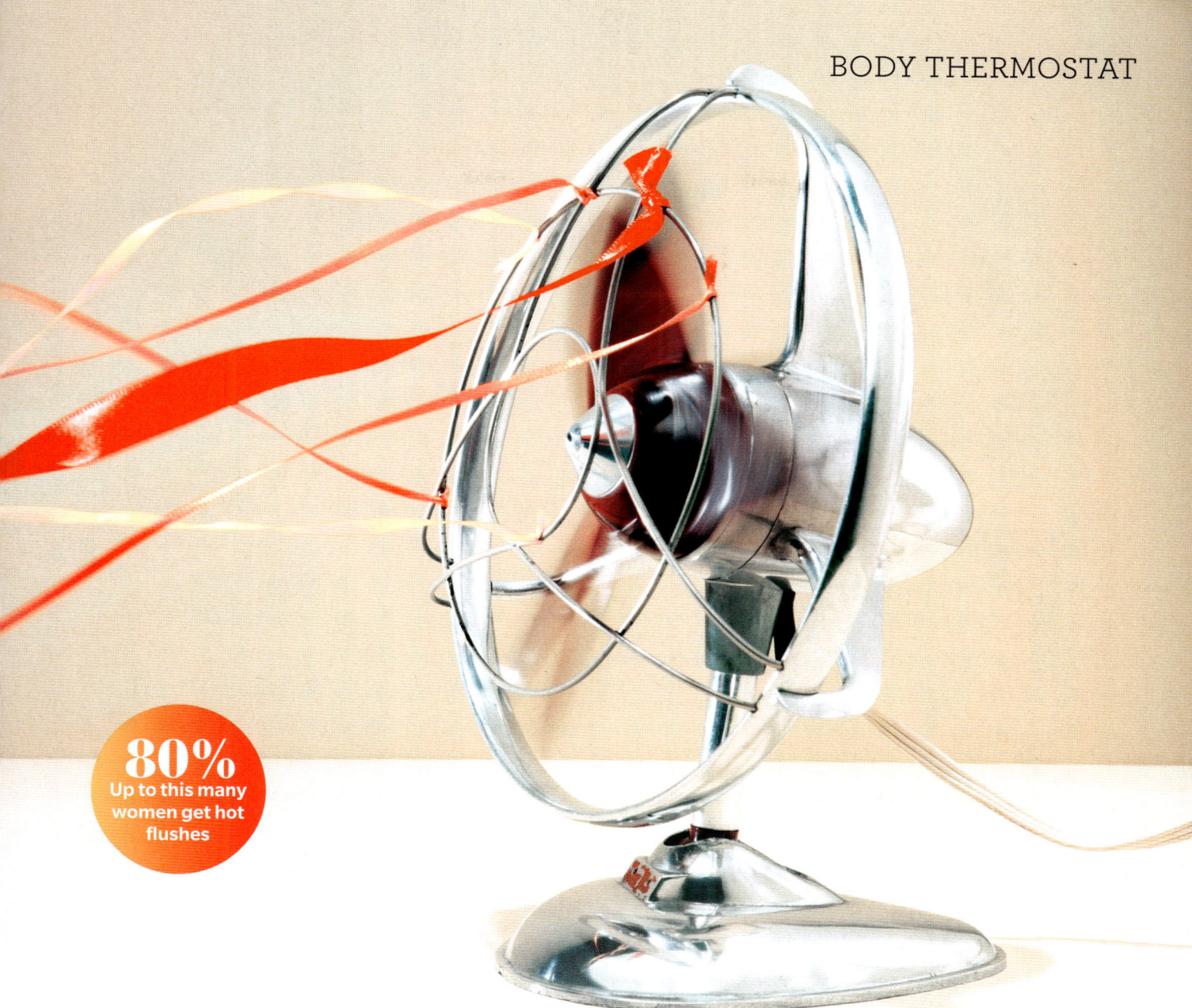

80% Up to this many women get hot flushes

Will herbs work for you?

The evidence: Many herbal remedies have been studied, such as red clover, ginseng, liquorice and black cohosh – on its own or with St John's wort. There's evidence the latter is effective for mild to moderate flushes and sleep-disrupting sweats.

How? It's not known exactly, but black cohosh may mimic oestrogen, and may also work on the parasympathetic nervous system. St John's wort helps to balance serotonin levels.

Try it: Pharmacies or health-food stores can suggest a supplement combining both herbs.

Note: Avoid if you've had breast cancer or liver disease. Stop taking it if you develop jaundice, dark urine or fatigue.

Put soya back on the menu

The evidence: It has long been speculated that soya quells flushes, but results have been mixed. However, a recent US analysis of 17 studies concluded that the equivalent of a couple of daily portions of soya-based foods and drinks lower frequency and severity of hot flushes by up to 26%.

How? Plant chemicals in soya, called isoflavones, are thought to mimic the effect of oestrogen.

Try it: You need 54mg of soya isoflavones daily for six weeks to a year. A serving of tofu (55g/2oz) or soya milk (600ml/1pt) contains 35-40mg of isoflavones.

Note: Try it for six weeks*. If there's no improvement, it could be that you don't produce equol, a substance produced by gut bacteria from soya foods. Non-equol producers don't benefit from soya.
*Try all remedies for at least six weeks, noting their efficacy.

The Smart Woman's Guide to the Menopause

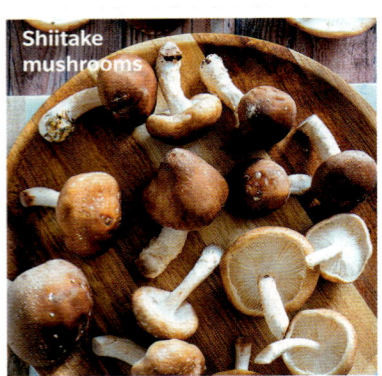
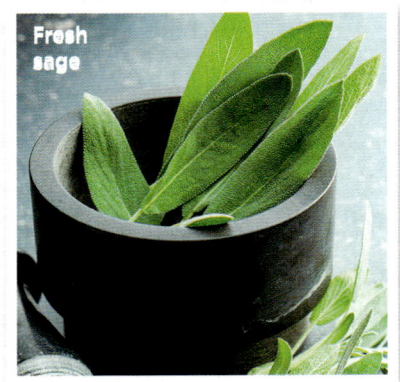
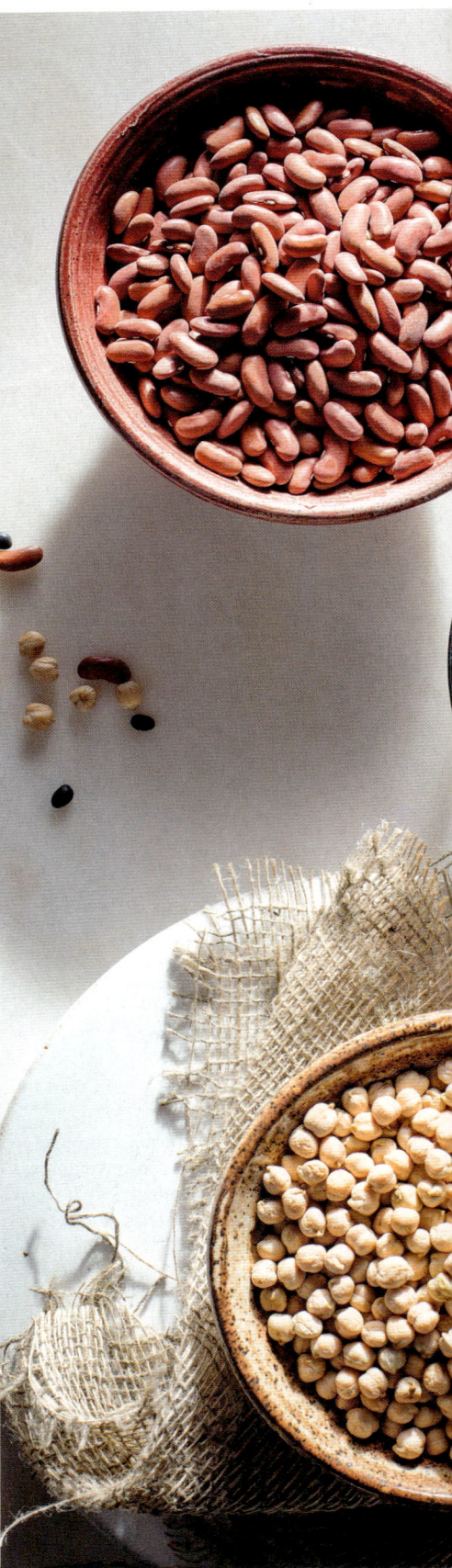

Eat foods that fight flushes

Nutritional therapist Nina Omotoso (nutritionwithnina.com) suggests five foods that help put a lid on those overheating episodes.

✦ **Flaxseed**
'Sprinkling flaxseed over cereal provides lignans, a type of plant oestrogen or phytoestrogen. During menopause, hormone levels can change quite rapidly,' says Nina. 'Phytoestrogens weakly imitate natural oestrogen activity, helping dampen down the effects of falling oestrogen and reducing the amount of hot flushes.' Try sprinkling some on your porridge.

✦ **Miso and tamari**
Derived from fermented soy beans, these Japanese foods are rich in isoflavones, a type of beneficial phytoestrogen. The fermentation process is key, says Nina.

✦ **Mushrooms**
Rich in the mineral selenium, which can help combat the mental and physical stress of hot flushes, shiitake mushrooms are used in Chinese medicine to alleviate menopause symptoms.
Nina's tip: 'Stir-fry mushrooms in tamari and lemon sprinkled with flaxseed, or thinly slice into miso soup.'

✦ **Sage**
'Research suggests that sage reduces both the severity and frequency of hot flushes and night sweats,' advises Nina. 'I often recommend sage tablets or sage tinctures, but also encourage my clients to drink sage tea or cook using the fresh herb as an ingredient.'

✦ **Beans and pulses**
'While they're also full of phytoestrogens, regularly eating these low-GL carbs can help keep your blood-glucose levels stable, preventing the dips that can trigger a hot flush,' says Nina.

BODY THERMOSTAT

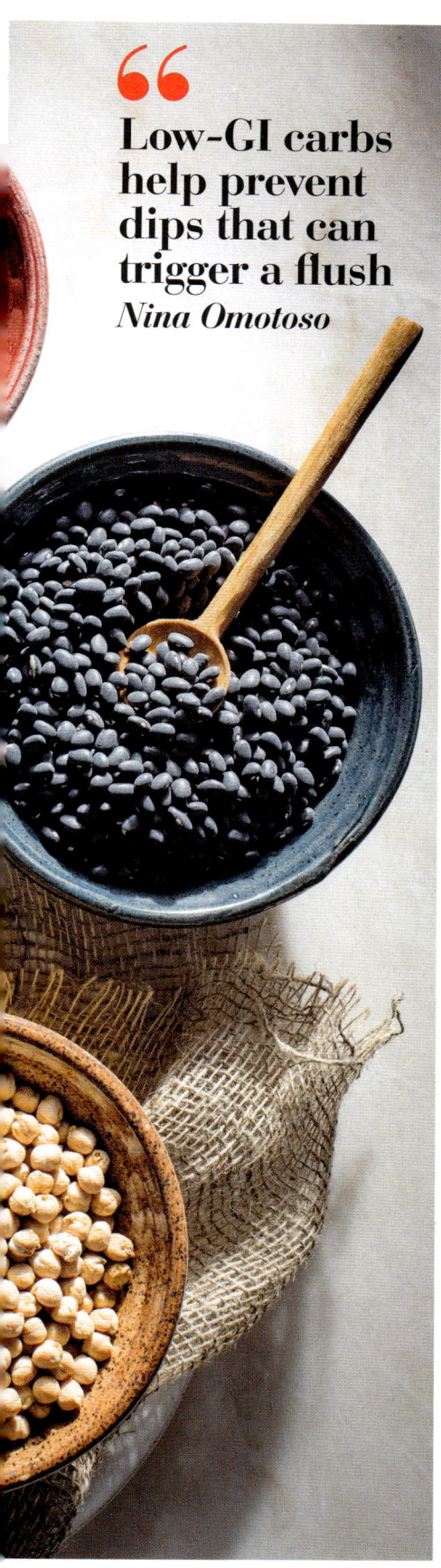

> Low-GI carbs help prevent dips that can trigger a flush
> Nina Omotoso

Book a course of acupuncture

The evidence: A study showed a course of acupuncture, twice a week for 10 weeks, reduced the severity, though not frequency, of hot flushes. Previous research has shown mixed results.
How? It's thought to alter the brain's mood chemistry by increasing endorphins. This in turn stabilises the body's temperature-control mechanism.
Try it: Find a local practitioner at The British Acupuncture Council (acupuncture.org.uk). The cost for a first consultation ranges from £45-£70, and £30-£50 per session thereafter.

Take a deep breath

The evidence: A technique called 'paced breathing' may shorten and cut down the number of flushes, according to a 2012 study from the Mayo clinic.
How? Slow, deep breathing is the fastest way to trigger into action your parasympathetic nervous system, which is involved in relaxing the muscles, slowing heart rate and lowering blood pressure.
Try it: Yoga or Pilates breathing is ideal – or follow this exercise: Find a quiet spot and breathe in deeply for five seconds. Now breathe out for another five seconds. Continue like this for 15 minutes and feel the warmth ebb away.

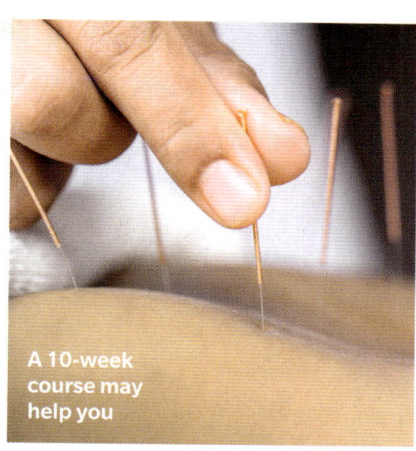

A 10-week course may help you

Keep your cool

Make sure the room is cool, and use a fan when a flush comes on. Spray your face with a cool-water atomiser, too, or use a cold gel pack (from pharmacies). Wear loose layers of light cotton or silk, and have layers of bed sheets instead of a duvet, so you can remove them as necessary. As a flush starts, sip a cold drink and have a lukewarm shower or bath.

Avoid triggers

Some foods can trigger or exacerbate hot flushes. They include alcohol, coffee, chocolate and spicy foods. 'These are stimulants that can aggravate hot flushes and night sweats in some women,' says dietitian Helen Bond. Oily fish, on the other hand, contains omega-3 fatty acids that may help reduce hot flushes.

5 QUICK FIXES

1 Australian Bush Flower Essences are natural remedies that can support your wellbeing. Try taking a few drops, morning and evening. Woman Bush Flower Essence, £11 for 30ml, nealsyardremedies.com.

2 If you find yourself constantly throwing off the duvet, having two single duvets rather than a double can solve the problem of your partner feeling the chill. Choose different weights to suit each of you and you should both sleep much better.

3 A fresh herbal tea will help to calm your flushes. Add 1-2tsp sage, motherwort or raspberry leaf to a cup of boiling water for five to 10 minutes, strain and drink. Buy herbs from baldwins.co.uk.

4 A cult buy for ladies who flush is the fantastic lightweight gel you smooth onto your skin to chill it instantly. Temple Spa Chillicious, £18 for 100ml, from victoriahealth.com.

5 The JML Chillmax Pillow, £11.99, boots.com, contains cooling gel to help you relax and sleep well. Pop it inside your pillowcase or rest your head on it directly for a chilled night's zzzs. Can also be used as a mat or a cushion.

The Smart Woman's Guide to the Menopause

The truth about HRT

HRT is surrounded by myths, so what's the truth? Charlotte Haigh examines the evidence and talks to the experts...

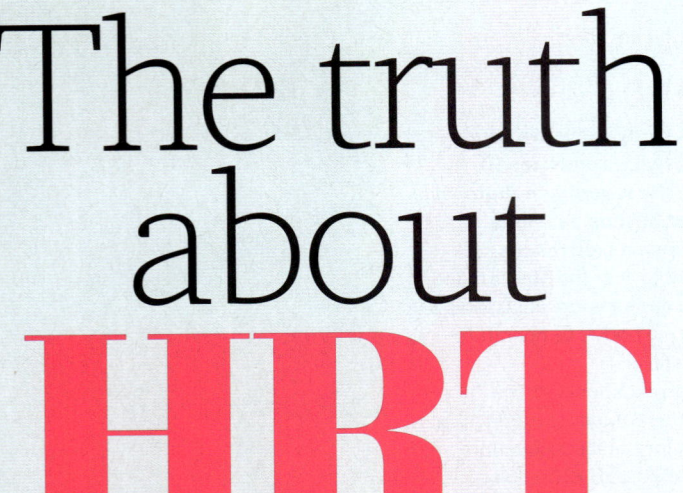

Recently, a friend in her late 40s rang me in tears. Her marriage was falling apart because she'd become so insecure and her husband couldn't cope. She kept having memory blanks during work meetings and her anxiety was so high she could no longer drive. Physically, she felt awful – her joints ached, her migraines had got worse and she'd put on weight because she no longer had energy to exercise. Her GP said she was perimenopausal and suggested HRT. 'But I'm not taking that stuff,' said my friend. 'I'd rather put up with this.'

Her take on HRT isn't unusual. Women in midlife have heard horror stories, and it's unsurprising they're sceptical, particularly as GPs don't always have the full facts.

A lot of the fears stem from a 2002 study, which raised concerns about the increased risk of breast cancer and heart disease. Subsequently, 50-70% of women stopped HRT. The research has since been found to be highly flawed, yet women still shun HRT – and that's sad when so many are suffering needlessly, says Dr Avrum Bluming, oncologist and co-author of *Oestrogen Matters* (£13.99, Piatkus).

So, what is the truth about HRT?

HEALTH REPORT

Won't I get menopause symptoms whenever I stop HRT?

'Some women do have symptoms when they stop HRT, but others find they don't come back,' says Dr Currie.

What's key is that you're likely to be in a very different life stage by then. You may start experiencing perimenopausal symptoms in your 40s when you're at the peak of your career and have teenagers at home – or even very young children, if you started a family later. You might be dating again after a divorce, getting into triathlons or starting up some new life projects.

Hot flushes, mood swings, anxiety and aching joints may really get in the way of your life at this age. If, however, you stave off symptoms with HRT until you're 60, you may be in a calmer phase of life – so, if symptoms do return, they may not have such a huge impact.

Declining oestrogen It drops to 1% of premenopause levels

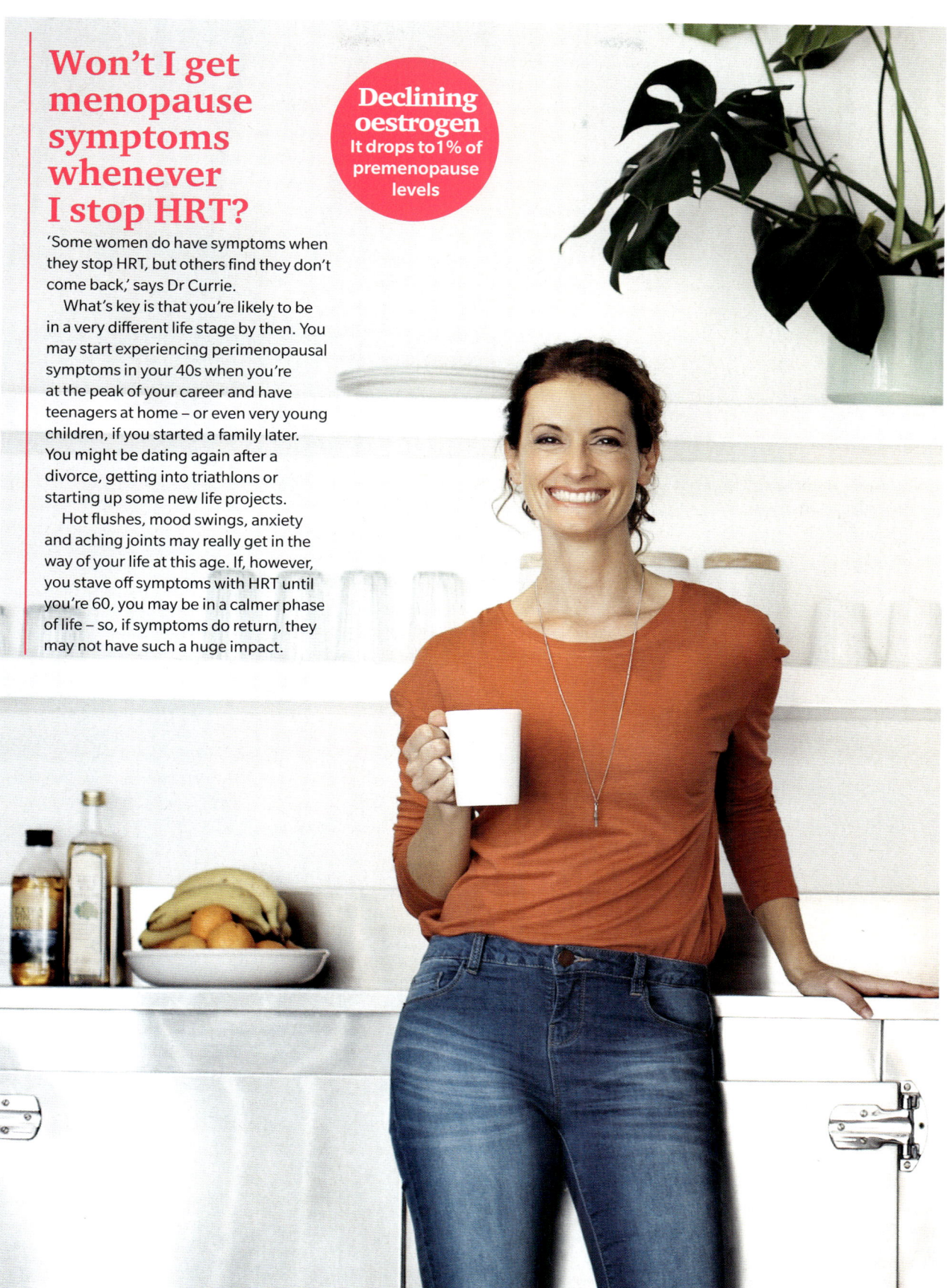

The Smart Woman's Guide to the Menopause

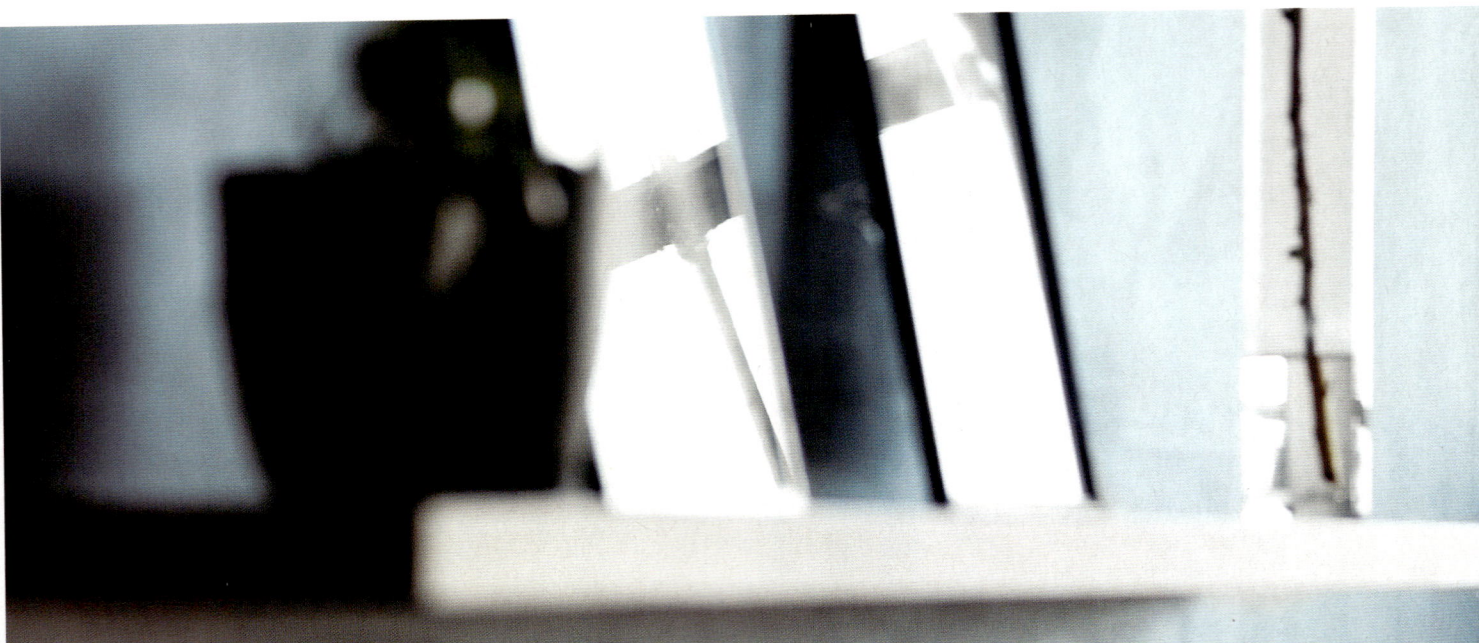

What exactly is HRT?

HRT is given in the form of supplementary hormones that replace what your body stops producing after menopause. Most women take a combination of oestrogen and progesterone, which both deplete as part of the body's natural changes.

If you have had a hysterectomy, you can take oestrogen without progesterone. Otherwise, taking oestrogen alone can raise your risk of womb cancer – and progesterone has been shown to reduce this risk.

HRT can be taken as pills, patches or in gel form. If you have perimenopausal symptoms but you're still having periods, your doctor will probably recommend cyclical HRT, which changes the dose throughout your cycle so you still get a bleed – that way, you'll know when your periods stop naturally.

> **HRT can quickly ease troublesome menopausal symptoms**
> *Dr Currie*

Are there other health benefits to HRT?

Yes. 'Firstly, it can quickly ease troublesome menopausal symptoms, such as hot flushes, vaginal dryness and anxiety, which can have a huge effect on your quality of life,' says Dr Heather Currie, gynaecologist and founder of menopausematters.co.uk.

But there may be longer-term health benefits, too. Dr Bluming explains that HRT is the only medicine proven to help slash the risk of dementia – by 45-60%. 'It is far superior to the small benefits from meditation or exercise, yet it's not well known.'

HRT has long been established as having a protective effect on bones. We lose up to 20% of our bone density in the five years after menopause. For this reason, NICE guidelines recommend any woman who goes through an early menopause (before the age of 45) should take HRT.

60% The amount by which HRT can cut the risk of dementia

What about the risk of heart disease and stroke?

This link also emerged from a WHI (Women's Health Initiative) study. But, of the women who took part in the research, many had existing heart risk factors. According to the BHF (British Heart Foundation), the latest research shows women taking HRT have no higher risk of dying from a heart attack or stroke than women who don't take it. In fact, some research – including a Danish study published in the *British Medical Journal* – found that HRT may actually have a protective effect on your cardiovascular health when started soon after menopause. Like any medicine, it isn't risk-free – oestrogen can cause platelets in the blood to clump, which may block arteries that are already narrowed. Your doctor can advise on your personal risk factors.

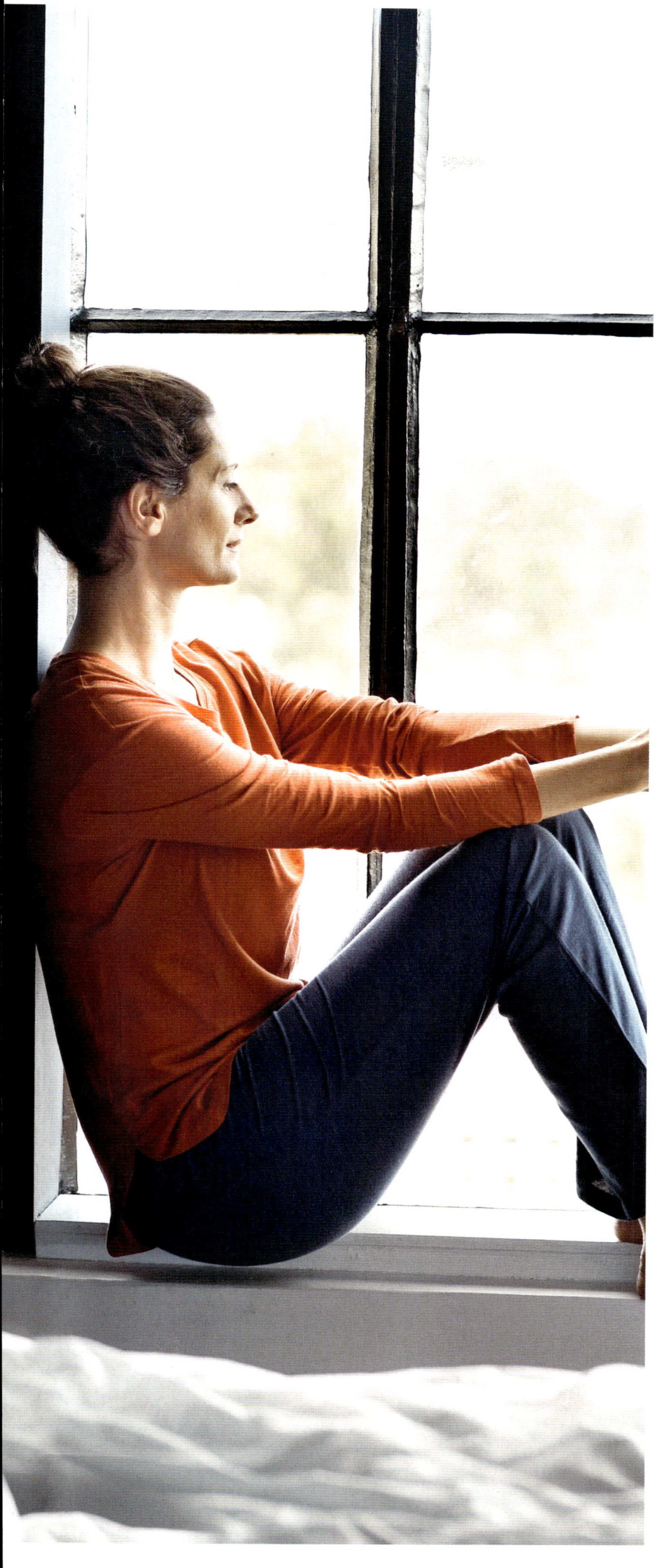

HEALTH REPORT

> It is far superior to the small benefits from meditation or exercise
>
> *Dr Bluming*

Doesn't HRT raise the risk of breast cancer?

Despite previous research showing HRT was safe, in 2002, the WHI study found it increased breast cancer risk. But Dr Bluming points out that what this actually amounted to was an extra eight cases of breast cancer for 10,000 women taking hormones for a year.

Bluming has looked at women genetically predisposed to breast cancer who'd had their ovaries removed before menopause, finding that their breast cancer risk fell by 50% when they were no longer exposed to oestrogen (which is produced in the ovaries). But, when these women were given replacement oestrogen after ovary removal, they still had the same lower risk of breast cancer. In other words, oestrogen isn't to blame.

'For the majority of women under 60 – and for some beyond that age – the benefits outweigh the risks of HRT,' says Dr Currie. 'Long-term use of a certain type of HRT after the age of 50 does carry a small increased risk of breast cancer – but being obese or drinking two units of alcohol a day both carry a greater risk.'

The Smart Woman's Guide to the Menopause

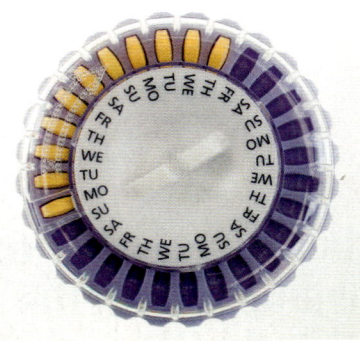

I still don't like the idea of it – isn't menopause a natural part of life?

It's important to remember our early ancestors would have died before – or shortly after – menopause. Now, because of increased lifespans, we're spending between a third to half our lives in oestrogen deficiency.

Dr Bluming's co-author, social psychologist Dr Carol Tavris, points out that, after menopause, oestrogen declines to only 1% of what it was, with effects on everything from mood, sleep and skin to bone density. Of course, not every woman has problems going through menopause – some breeze through with few symptoms. But, if it's affecting your quality of life or relationships – or if you go through it young – it's important to have the full picture when you're making a decision.

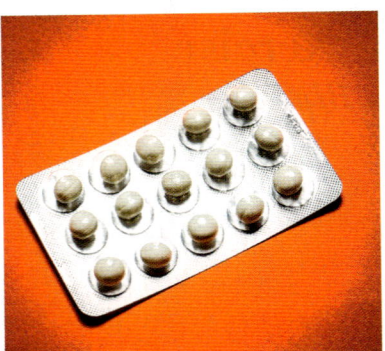

Can I try bioidentical hormones if I want a more natural approach?

There's a lot of misunderstanding about bioidentical hormones, which can be prescribed privately. Although they're derived from plant sources, they're still processed, and the resulting hormones are a little different to those found in standard HRT.

Some women prefer bioidentical hormones because they can be tailored, but there's currently no evidence that there's any advantage to this type of HRT. There are definitely good reasons to talk to your doctor about different types of HRT, though. For example, Premarin, which is derived from pregnant mares' urine, is still routinely prescribed, and you may have ethical concerns about using this, particularly if you're vegan.

Fortunately, there are alternative forms of HRT, so do have an open conversation with your doctor. If you decide against HRT, there are ways you can manage symptoms with herbs and nutrition. **A.Vogel Menopause Support** is a good place to start: avogel.co.uk/health/menopause.

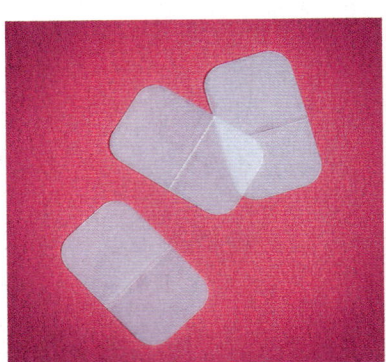

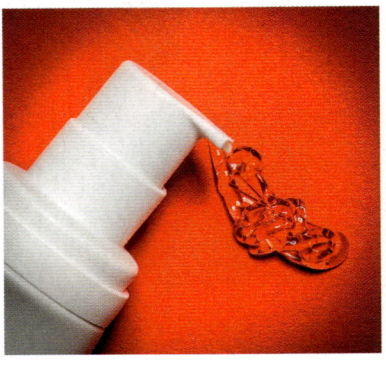

Busting HRT myths
The experts reveal the facts

✦ **HRT causes clots**
'If you take oral (tablet) HRT, there's a small increased risk of a clot developing in your legs or lungs,' says Dr Louise Newson, GP and menopause specialist (menopausedoctor.co.uk). 'This increased risk is very small, but is heightened by risk factors, including obesity or a history of clots. However, if you take the oestrogen part of HRT as either a gel or patch, then it gets absorbed directly into your body, which means the clotting factors in your liver aren't activated [which they are when you swallow a tablet].'

✦ **HRT interrupts the menopause**
'This is not true – you can't stop and start the menopause, that's not how the body works,' says Jane Atherton, clinical nutritionist, menopause lifestyle coach and member of the British Menopause Society. 'HRT will help relieve symptoms while you're taking it,' she explains, adding, 'If symptoms return when you stop, this is what your body would have done regardless. It doesn't mean you have gone back to the beginning of your menopause.'

✦ **I can only use HRT for a limited time**
'There's no fixed time limit on how long you can use HRT, although most women will only need to use it for two to three years,' explains Dr Kathryn Basford, GP at online doctor Zava. Plus, some risks associated with HRT can increase the longer it's used for. 'Your doctor should review your prescription annually to ensure the type of HRT you're on is still suitable,' adds Dr Newson.

FASHION

Her light materials

Game changers
New fabrics to keep you dry

The right fabrics can make a real difference when you have a hot flush or night sweat. Lisa Buckingham has some suggestions...

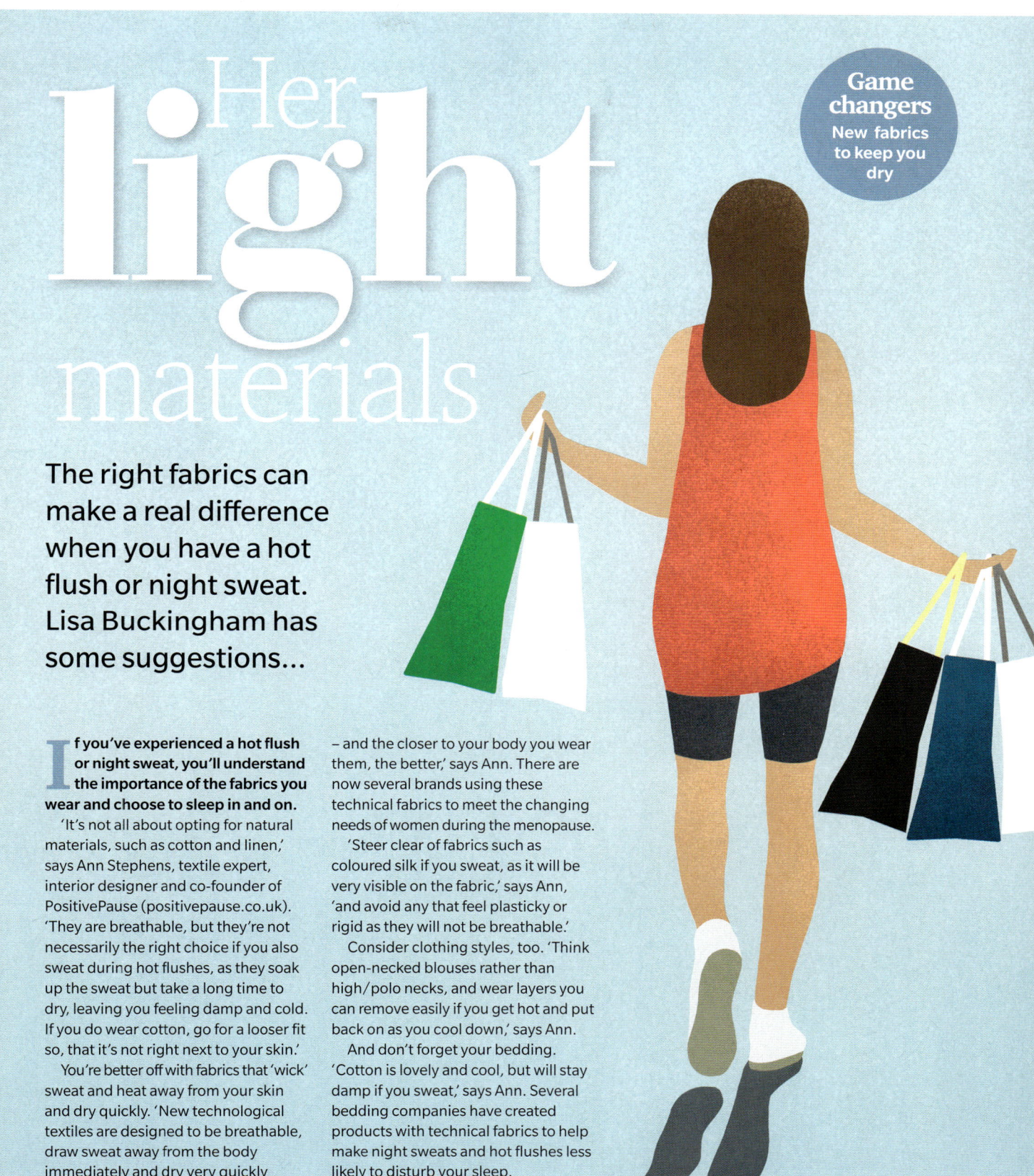

If you've experienced a hot flush or night sweat, you'll understand the importance of the fabrics you wear and choose to sleep in and on.

'It's not all about opting for natural materials, such as cotton and linen,' says Ann Stephens, textile expert, interior designer and co-founder of PositivePause (positivepause.co.uk). 'They are breathable, but they're not necessarily the right choice if you also sweat during hot flushes, as they soak up the sweat but take a long time to dry, leaving you feeling damp and cold. If you do wear cotton, go for a looser fit so, that it's not right next to your skin.'

You're better off with fabrics that 'wick' sweat and heat away from your skin and dry quickly. 'New technological textiles are designed to be breathable, draw sweat away from the body immediately and dry very quickly – and the closer to your body you wear them, the better,' says Ann. There are now several brands using these technical fabrics to meet the changing needs of women during the menopause.

'Steer clear of fabrics such as coloured silk if you sweat, as it will be very visible on the fabric,' says Ann, 'and avoid any that feel plasticky or rigid as they will not be breathable.'

Consider clothing styles, too. 'Think open-necked blouses rather than high/polo necks, and wear layers you can remove easily if you get hot and put back on as you cool down,' says Ann.

And don't forget your bedding. 'Cotton is lovely and cool, but will stay damp if you sweat,' says Ann. Several bedding companies have created products with technical fabrics to help make night sweats and hot flushes less likely to disturb your sleep.

Exercise matters

Like muscles, our skeleton becomes stronger when we exercise. 'It can help delay the rate of age-related bone loss,' explains Craig Sale, professor of human physiology at Nottingham Trent University. 'But stick to exercise that uses your body weight, alongside weight resistance exercise (such as strength training). Even the easiest of movements can boost bones. Try gentle press-ups against a wall to strengthen wrists and for hips, stand on one leg for one minute, three times a day.

One in three menopausal women suffer from osteoporosis. Our tips will help strengthen your skeleton and reduce your risk…

Give your bones a boost →

BONE HEALTH

Did you know that you have 206 bones in your body? And all of them play a vital role. But, during and after the menopause, women lose essential bone mass or density, which can play havoc with your health.

'This is why one in three menopausal women will suffer osteoporosis compared with one in five men as we age,' says pharmacologist Dr Omar Milhem. 'It happens because oestrogen plays a pivotal role in regulating bone balance. When oestrogen is withdrawn from the female body during menopause, this increases an internal inflammatory response to break down more bone at an accelerated rate.'

And, if you don't try to prevent your bones deteriorating, it could affect your mobility in older age, with stats revealing that one in two women over 50 will break a bone. You'll have a diagnosis of osteoporosis if you've lost a significant amount of bone, but you may not even realise you have it until you break a bone during a minor fall or accident.

'Overall, the bones become more brittle and may break more easily,' says Dr Milhem. 'The spine becomes more compressed as vertebrae lose mineral content, making each bone thinner. As a result, posture may become more stooped, knees and hips may become more flexed, and shoulders may narrow, while the pelvis becomes wider.'

But the good news is you can reduce and delay the onset or progression of osteoporosis and boost your bone health. Here's how…

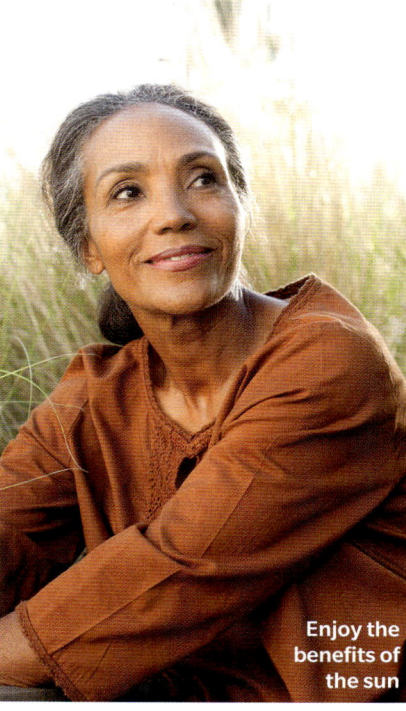
Enjoy the benefits of the sun

Get outside

The Royal Osteoporosis Society suggests a 10-minute stroll outside once or twice a day to boost the body's vitamin D.

'Without sufficient levels, you can't absorb key ingredients, leading to poor bone mineralisation and increased risk of osteoporosis,' says Dr Sarah Brewer.

This is particularly critical for perimenopausal women. The ability to synthesise vitamin D through your skin drops for the over-50s by four times.

'I believe that most adults would benefit from 25mcg per day, increasing to 50mcg

Reduce salt intake

The more salt consumed, the more calcium is lost. 'Just 2,300mg of sodium takes out 40mg of calcium, potentially exacerbating the risk of osteoporosis,' says nutritionist Shane Bilsborough.

The body does need a certain ratio of sodium to potassium for optimal bone health but, when sodium intake rises, there's an imbalance. So, while cheese is a great source of calcium, watch out which ones you choose.

'Those high in salt, like Roquefort, Parmesan, feta and processed cheese, aren't so beneficial,' says Professor Susan Lanham-New, head of nutritional sciences at the University of Surrey.

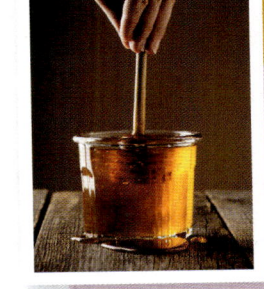

Love honey

Scientists at Purdue University in the US found honey may help the body to absorb calcium more effectively. 'The minerals found in honey include calcium, copper, iron and magnesium,' says orthopaedic surgeon Raja Ahluwalia. 'And in laboratory studies, it's been shown to increase the absorption of calcium from the gut.'

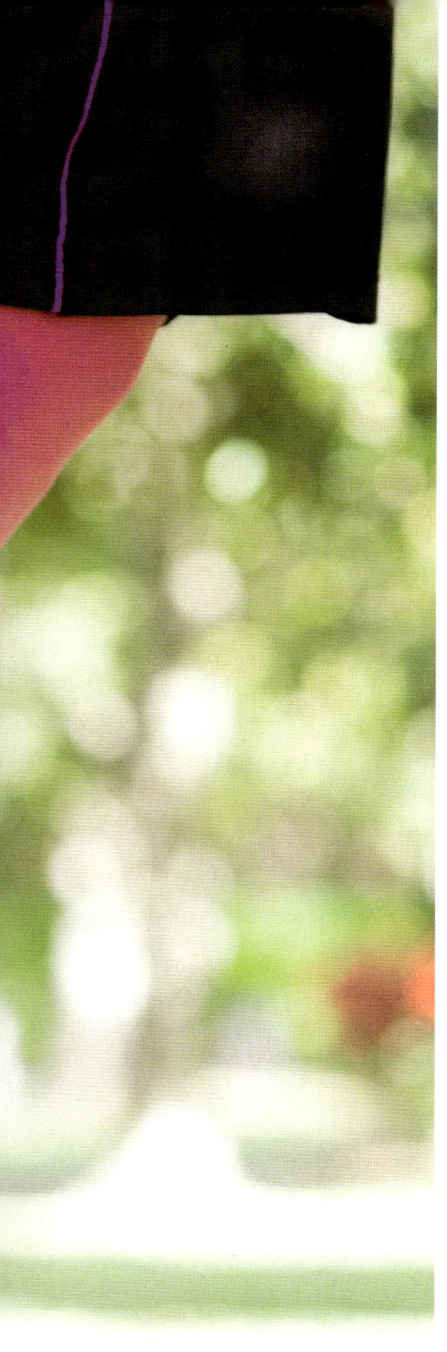

> " If you have lost height, or are worried, ask your GP about a bone density scan

The Smart Woman's Guide to the Menopause 37

from 50 onwards,' says Dr Brewer. Try **Fultium Daily D3, £3.99 for 30 capsules.**

See your GP
If you've noticed you are losing height or developing a stoop, your GP can assess if you're at risk of developing osteoporosis. It may be due to compression fractures in the spine caused by fragile bones. Worried? Speak to your doctor about having a bone mineral density (DEXA) scan.

Check your medications
'A number of medications, such as steroids, have a negative effect on bone metabolism and can induce osteoporosis,' says Mr Ahluwalia, consultant orthopaedic surgeon at The Lister Hospital, part of HCA Healthcare UK (hcahealthcare.co.uk).

'These medications allow the treatment of conditions that have a strong inflammatory response, such as rheumatoid arthritis and lupus. Their use can make the bone brittle and lead to fractures or breaks at low forces – such as a fall from standing height. Other medications, such as aspirin, also inhibit bone healing.'

Never stop taking your medication, but ask your GP about ways to lower the risks.

Stub it out
A study by the Feinberg School of Medicine in Chicago found smokers with specific bone injuries took two months longer to heal than non-smokers. This is because nicotine constricts blood vessels, so fewer nutrients are supplied to the bones.

'The evidence linking smoking with increased fracture risk is so strong, it is a scientifically validated risk factor included in FRAX (the World Health Organisation's fracture risk assessment tool), which calculates an individual's 10-year risk of osteoporotic fracture,' says Mr Ahluwalia.

The best thing you can do for your bones is to quit, even later in life it can help limit smoking-related bone loss.

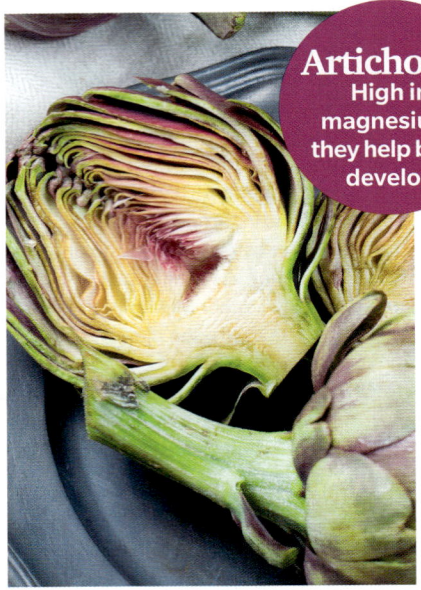

Artichokes High in magnesium, they help bone develop

Tuck into artichokes
Each one contains 72mg of skeleton-supporting magnesium and 425mg of potassium. Magnesium is an abundant mineral in the human body, with 50-60% found in bones. It's necessary for the structural development of bone and ensuring the parathyroid glands, which produce hormones important for bone health, work normally.

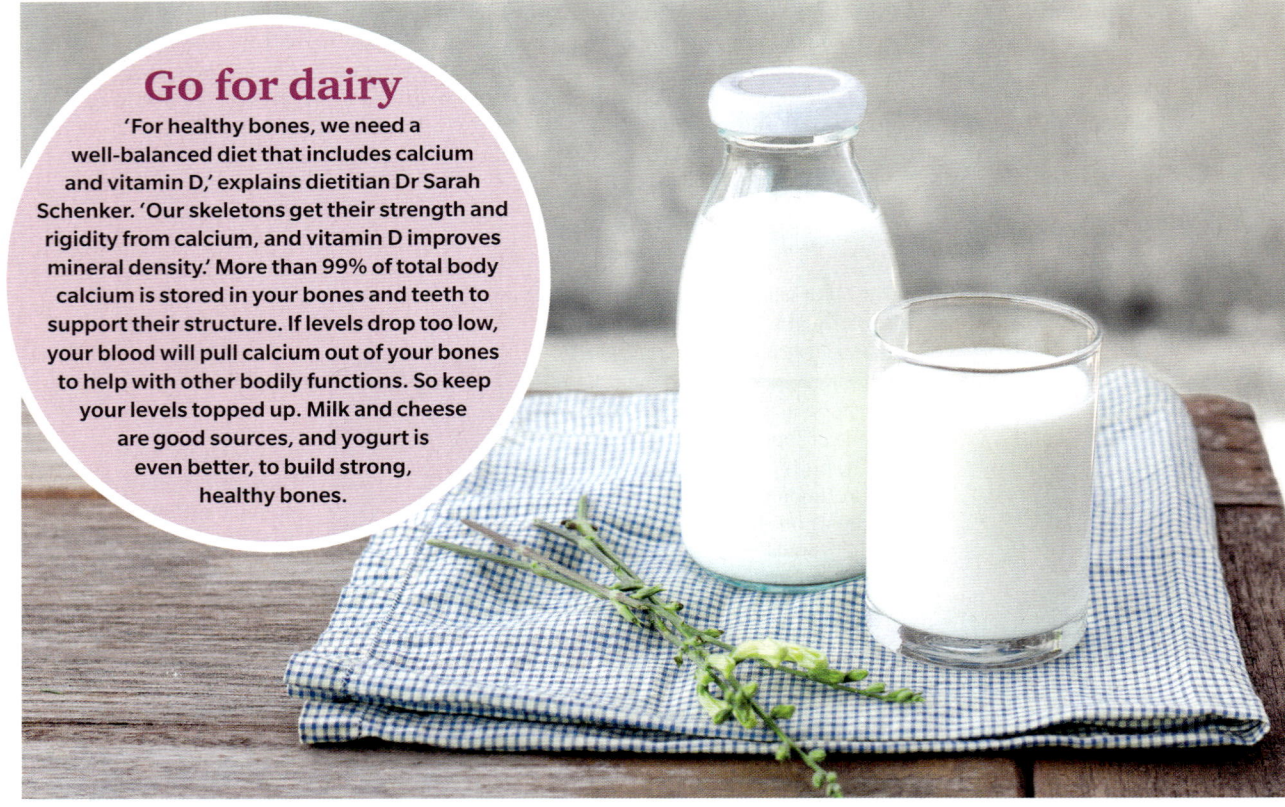

Go for dairy
'For healthy bones, we need a well-balanced diet that includes calcium and vitamin D,' explains dietitian Dr Sarah Schenker. 'Our skeletons get their strength and rigidity from calcium, and vitamin D improves mineral density.' More than 99% of total body calcium is stored in your bones and teeth to support their structure. If levels drop too low, your blood will pull calcium out of your bones to help with other bodily functions. So keep your levels topped up. Milk and cheese are good sources, and yogurt is even better, to build strong, healthy bones.

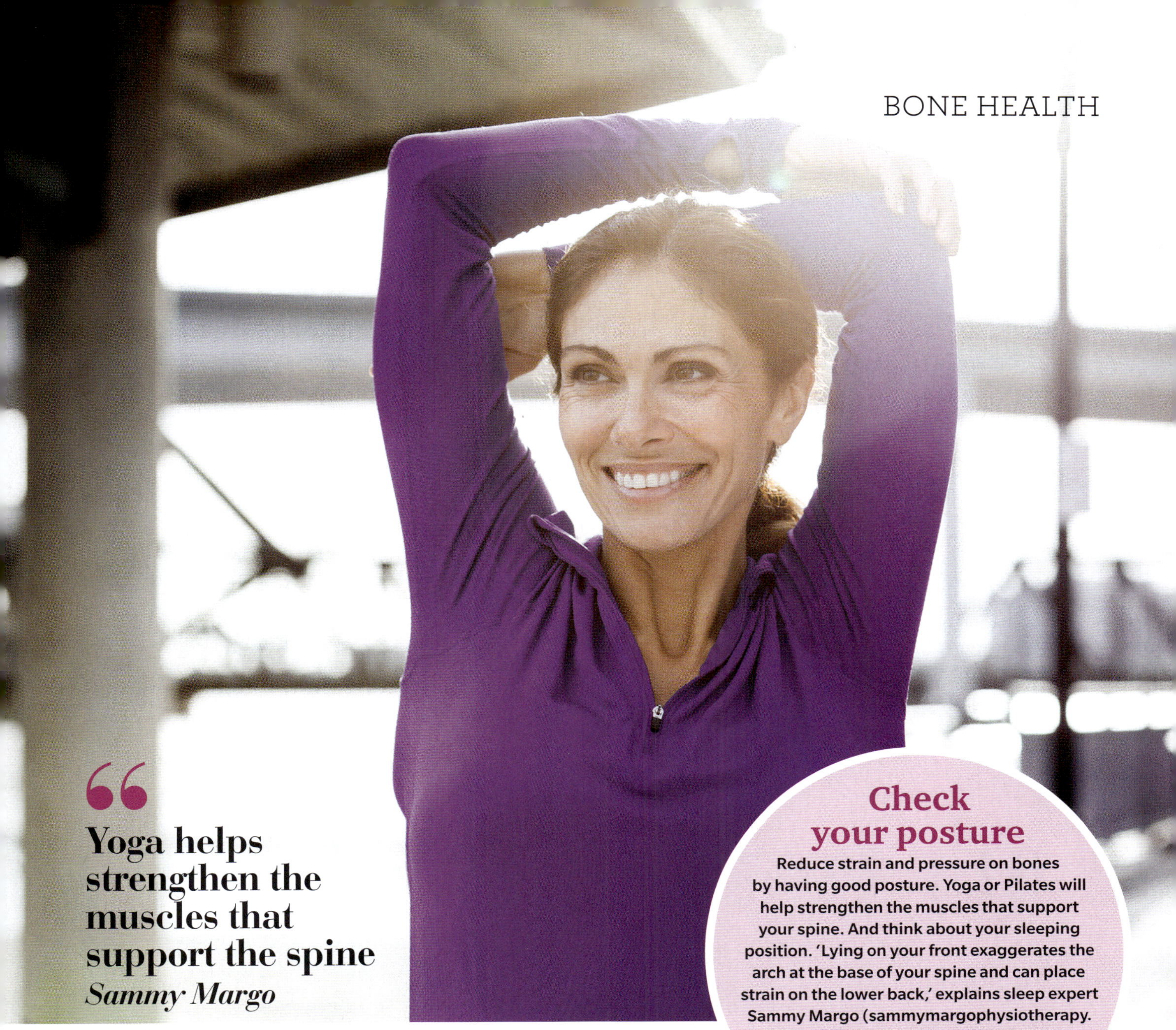

BONE HEALTH

> **Yoga helps strengthen the muscles that support the spine**
> *Sammy Margo*

Have your prunes
'A recent study found that postmenopausal women who ate 10 prunes a day had significantly higher bone density than a control group who ate only apples,' says naturopathic nutritionist Amy Morris.

This bone strengthening is thanks to antioxidants called polyphenols, which help to slow down the rate of bone loss.

'Prunes are also high in vitamin K, great for the connective tissue that makes up bones,' says physiotherapist Tim Allardyce.

Can the cola
'Phosphoric acid in carbonated beverages can cause an increase in the acidity levels of blood,' says Amy. 'This causes the body to pull calcium out of bones to bring down the acidity levels.'

Get fruity
We all know oranges are packed with vitamin C, but did you know that this forms collagen in the bones, which acts like a glue to keep calcium where it's needed? Bananas and kiwi fruit are full of potassium, while plums contain a fibre called inulin, which helps calcium absorption. But watch out. 'Fruit is packed with sugars,' warns Tim. 'So don't be tempted to overfill your diet with fruit.'

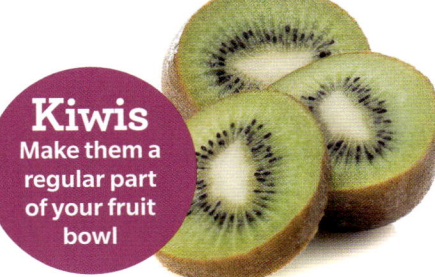

Kiwis Make them a regular part of your fruit bowl

Check your posture
Reduce strain and pressure on bones by having good posture. Yoga or Pilates will help strengthen the muscles that support your spine. And think about your sleeping position. 'Lying on your front exaggerates the arch at the base of your spine and can place strain on the lower back,' explains sleep expert Sammy Margo (sammymargophysiotherapy.com). 'Maintain the spine's natural curves by side-sleeping, or sleeping on your back with a pillow placed under your knees.'

Avoid going on a crash diet
Being a healthy weight is best for your bones, as being overweight or obese can put unnecessary stress on your body, especially the knee joints. If you need to lose weight though, do so in a sustainable way.

'Crash diets bring with them a possible reduction of bone mineral density and an increased risk of developing osteoporosis,' says Jonathan Tobias, Professor of rheumatology at Bristol University.

The Smart Woman's Guide to the Menopause

Save your skin

Fluctuating hormones can wreak havoc on your complexion. It's time to fight back with our skin SOS guide

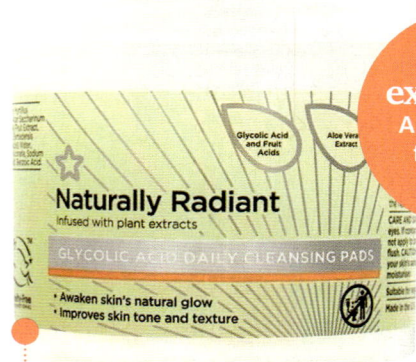

Gentle exfoliation A sure way to freshen up your face

Get a glow
Face looking grey and lacklustre? That's due to a build up of dead skin cells, which leaves your complexion looking dull. The solution? Gentle exfoliation at least twice a week to sweep them away and freshen up your face. Try **Superdrug Naturally Radiant Glycolic Acid Daily Cleansing Pads, £6.99,** which can be used every day if you wish.

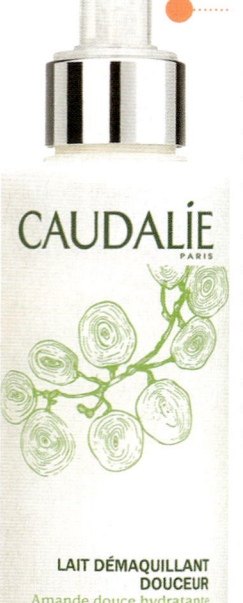

Rehydrate parched skin
Our skin starts to lose the ability to hold water after menopause, which can leave it feeling dry and looking flaky. Use a mild cleanser that won't strip your skin of moisture. We love **Caudalie Gentle Cleansing Milk, £9, lookfantastic.com**, which is enriched with soothing, hydrating ingredients.

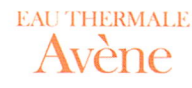
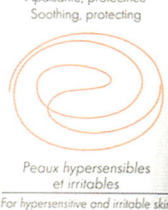

Calm irritation
If your skin has suddenly become ultra-sensitive, simplify your care regime pronto. Look out for sensitive, skin-friendly products that are soothing and fragrance-free. Try **Avène Skin Recovery Cream, £16.50, Boots,** which contains an ingredient called parcerine to quickly calm irritation.

SKINCARE

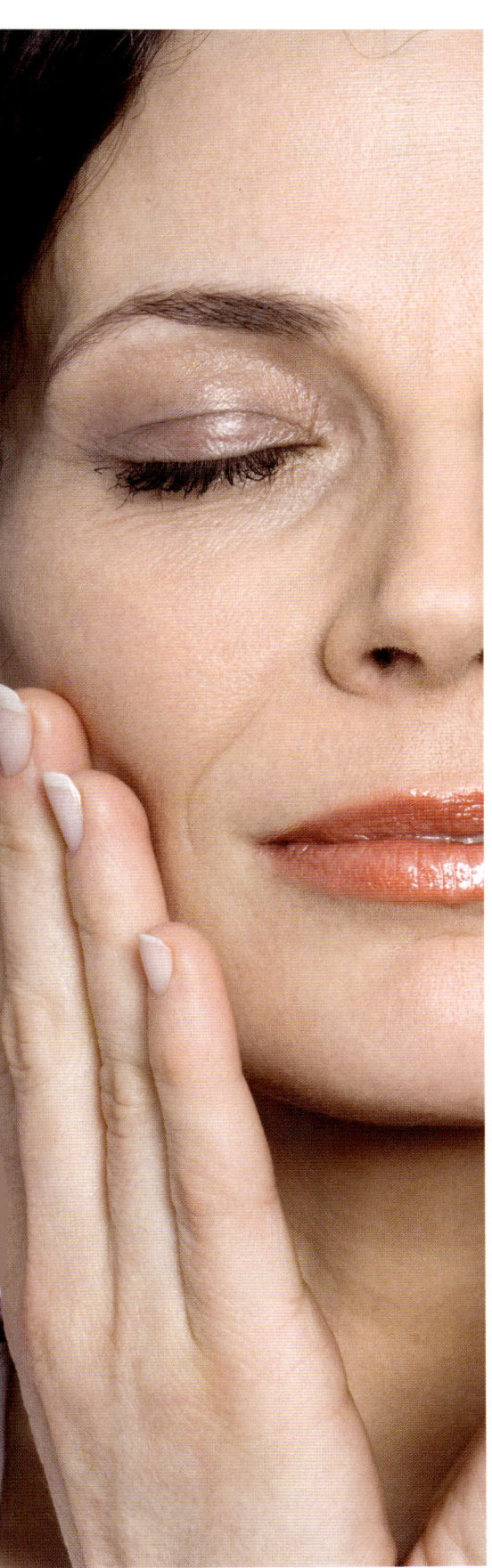

Zap spots
Spots can be a problem during and after menopause. Use face washes and moisturisers that contain salicylic acid, glycolic acid or niacinamide to destroy bacteria and reduce inflammation. Try **Super Facialist Salicylic Acid Purifying Cleansing Wash, £9.**

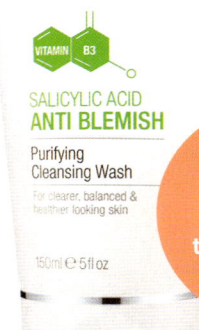

Wash carefully Kill bacteria that can cause blemishes

Prevent pigmentation
Our skin is more at risk from UV damage after the menopause. That's because the levels of melanin, the pigment that protects our skin from the sun, starts to reduce. Prevent damage by using a moisturiser with SPF every single day. Try **Alpha-H Essential Skin Perfecting Moisturiser SPF15, £29, lookfantastic.com,** which shields from UV damage and pollution.

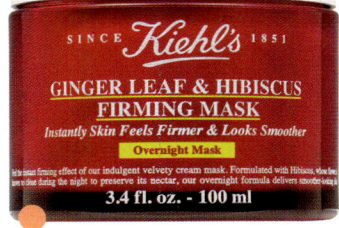

Blitz facial hair
The menopause can cause a surge in testosterone, which, for some, can cause hair to sprout on the chin. Instead of plucking stragglers, use a dermaplaner – a slim, stainless steel blade – to remove unwanted hair. We also love the **Hollywood Browzer, £8.95, hollywoodbrowzer.com,** which will whisk hair away.

Tighten up sagging
Collagen and elastin levels in our skin drop dramatically after we hit menopause, causing wrinkles and sagging. Forget the facelift, **Kiehl's Ginger Leaf & Hibiscus Firming Mask, £44,** may be pricey but it's a game changer.

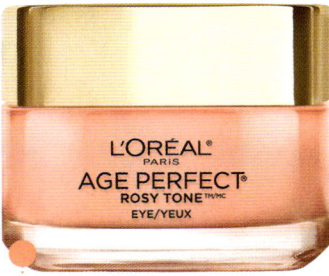

Brighten tired eyes
Whether it's night sweats or insomnia, if you're not sleeping the circulation around our eyes get sluggish. Use a cream like **L'Oréal Paris Age Perfect Golden Age Rosy Radiant Eye Cream, £14.99,** to reduce dark circles.

Soothe flushing
Suffering from hot flushes and/or red, sensitive skin? Calm with a cooling mask. **REN Evercalm Ultra Comforting Rescue Mask, £32, lookfantastic.com,** quickly neutralises redness in the skin and soothes dryness. Use it to give your skin a boost.

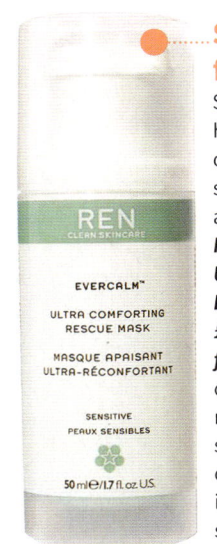

The Smart Woman's Guide to the Menopause

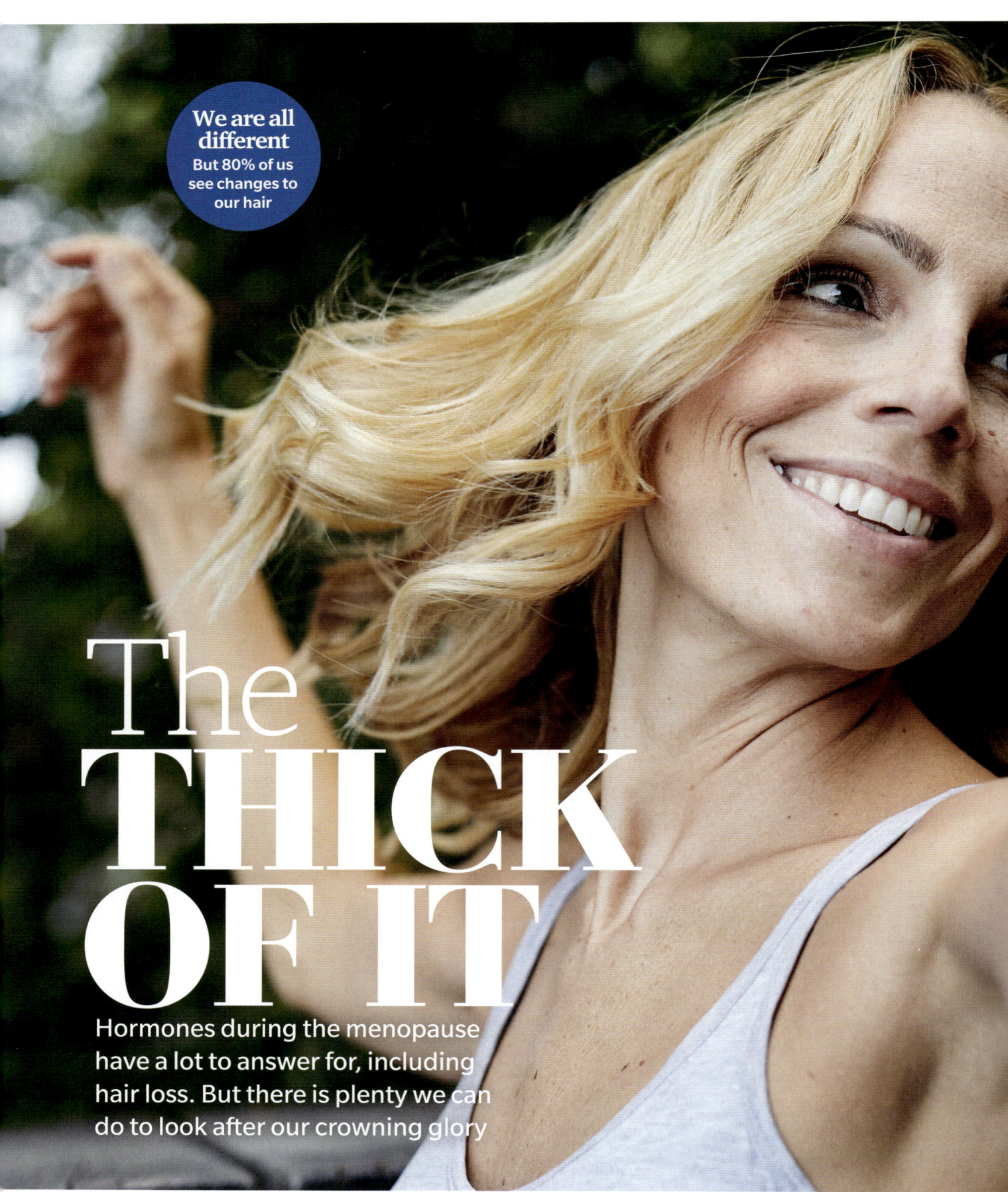

We are all different But 80% of us see changes to our hair

The THICK OF IT

Hormones during the menopause have a lot to answer for, including hair loss. But there is plenty we can do to look after our crowning glory

HAIR LOSS

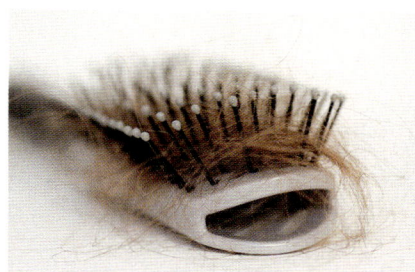

During the menopause, as our hormones are all over the place, 40% of women will suffer from thinning hair. As oestrogen decreases, it shortens the growth cycle so hair doesn't grow as long. Plus the menopause increases androgens (the male hormone), which affects the thickness of each strand.

'The changes that occur to hair during the menopause can shatter confidence,' says hairdresser Debbie Ford. 'I've had women come to me in tears with thinning hair and bald patches. Every woman is different, but around 80% will experience changes to the volume and texture of their hair as a result of hormonal shifts during perimenopause and menopause. As hormone levels decrease, hair gets more brittle, less bouncy and there is inevitably a certain amount of hair loss.'

Thinning hair can create a lot of anxiety, but there are things you can do to get it looking great again.

Is my hair thinning?

There are seven early signs to look out for, say the trichology experts at Philip Kingsley.

✦ Your hair is shedding more than is normal for you for longer than two months. You'll notice more hair fall than usual when you shampoo, when you brush your hair and perhaps on your pillow and clothes. Also, if you leave more days between shampooing than you usually do, the amount of hair falling out that you see will be more noticeable.

✦ You feel your ponytail is thinner than it once was.

✦ Your scalp is becoming more visible and/or you notice a reduction in overall volume or density.

✦ You find your hair is unable to grow as long as it used to.

✦ Your ends are finer than they used to be, yet they are not breaking. In this instance, you may notice many new hairs of different lengths growing from your scalp.

✦ You notice that your hair is gradually becoming finer at the front, crown or temple regions of your scalp.

✦ You notice excessive growth of hair on other parts of your body, such as your face, chest or arms.

THICKER HAIR HEROES

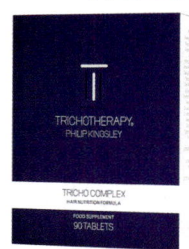 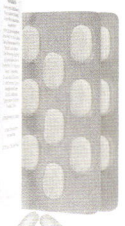

Breakfast boost
Philip Kingsley Tricho Complex Food Supplement, £45 for 90 tablets, philipkingsley.co.uk, contain hair-loving vitamins and minerals. Take two at breakfast daily for four months.

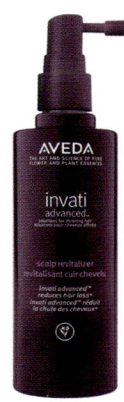

Treat your scalp
Taking care of your scalp will boost healthy hair. *Aveda Invati Scalp Revitalizer, £49, aveda.co.uk*, uses special herbs to stimulate the scalp and boost circulation so hair loss is minimised.

Pump up the volume
Prep just-washed hair with *Swell Ultimate Volume Root Complex, £32, swell.co.uk*, before styling. It feeds your roots, so over time you'll see less shedding, and injects volume for a fuller blow-dry.

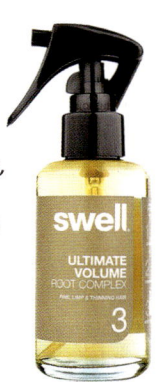

Do the double
Dry shampoo is a lifesaver when there's no time to wash your hair. *Bouffe Professional Hair Thickening Spray, £12.50,* goes one better by bulking up fine, thin hair so it looks bigger and thicker. It even comes in different shades to cover grey regrowth.

FEED YOUR HAIR

The right diet can work wonders, but it may take anything from three to six months to see a marked improvement.

✦ Eat more fresh vegetables and fruit: have 5-10 (80g) portions every day.
✦ Eat oily fish at least twice a week.
✦ Choose good-quality meat.
✦ Include protein with every meal.
✦ Eat healthy fats. Pumpkin, sunflower and flax seeds are especially good. And try avocados and nuts. We love *Waitrose Mixed Nuts, Fruit & Seeds, £1*.
✦ Avoid low-fat products.
✦ Vitamin B12, zinc and biotin are crucial for healthy hair. Eggs and sweet potatoes are a good source of biotin, and seafood contains zinc. Beef, liver, chicken, eggs, yogurt and cheese contain vitamin B12.
✦ Take a nutritional supplement. Try *Viviscal Maximum Strength Hair Growth Supplement, £38.99 for 60 tablets*.
✦ Keep blood-sugar levels balanced by eating regularly.
✦ Avoid having alcohol, caffeine and processed foods.

Other reasons for hair loss

STRESS In extreme circumstances, feeling anxious can cause hair loss.
GENETICS Sadly, if one or both of your parents suffered hair loss, you could inherit the same gene.
DIET Healthy hair starts from the inside out. Aim for a mix of protein and iron, plus fruit and veg.
HEALTH Polycystic ovaries, thyroid problems, some meds and general poor health can cause hair loss.

The Smart Woman's Guide to the Menopause

DID YOU KNOW? Sit-ups can actually put pressure on a weak pelvic floor and lead to a prolapsed bladder or uterus

Your complete guide to a
STRONGER
pelvic floor

BLADDER ISSUES

Incontinence problems are more common than we'd like to admit. Here's how to deal with them

Do you dread running, jumping, coughing or sneezing because you might wet yourself? Sadly, you're not alone – especially once you have been through the menopause. Yet many women are living with restricted lives and daily embarrassment, which could be sorted out if they asked for some help.

The floor of our pelvis is made up of muscles and other tissues, which stretch from the tailbone at the back to the pubic bone in front. Not only do these muscles support our bladder, uterus, colon, vagina and anus – they literally keep everything in – but they are also responsible for some of our vital bodily functions.

'They support our posture and physical movements, as well as helping with bowel and bladder control and sexual function,' explains Pilates and postnatal fitness expert Jane Wake.

But, like any other muscle, sometimes our pelvic floor isn't as strong as it should be. A weakened pelvic floor can cause a loss of bladder control, which often results in stress incontinence – women may leak small amounts of urine when they cough, sneeze or exercise.

It can also cause other symptoms, such as failing to reach the loo in time, uncontrollably breaking wind, reduced sensation in the vagina, a distinct bulge at the vaginal opening and a heavy sensation in the vagina.

Our pelvic floor can be weakened by pregnancy, birth, being overweight, chronic constipation, constant coughing, as well as some forms of surgery.

But one of the most common causes is the menopause. 'Decreasing hormones are the biggest reason as to why women in the peri and menopausal stages of life will have issues,' explains Jane. 'Both the male sex hormone testosterone and the female hormone oestrogen play a major role in maintaining and promoting muscle integrity. 'As these hormones lower, muscles can lose connection and strength, leading to issues, such as incontinence and pelvic weakness.'

Tone up Strengthen the pelvic floor regularly

Get a boost

'To effectively train a weakened pelvic floor, you need to be aiming for at least 100 contractions daily,' explains Jane.

Tired just thinking about it? **Innovo shorts (£324.99 for the starter kit, myinnovo.com)** could be your saviour. They look like an ordinary pair of cycling shorts, but with built-in electrical pads. Slip them on and non-invasive NMES technology stimulates your pelvic-floor muscles, enabling 180 contractions of the pelvic floor in just 30 minutes.

Perfect pads

Feel confident and safer when it comes to leaks, thanks to these knickers with benefits…
♦ For every day: *Pretty Clever Pants (from £16.99 for two, prettycleverpants.com).* Designed by TV presenter Carol Smillie, these look just like normal knickers.
♦ For ultra absorbency: *Intime Super (£14.99, id-direct.com).* Absorb eight times their own weight for maximum protection.
♦ For something special: *Tena Silhouette Noir (£8, Boots).* Designed to help women feel sexy, despite incontinence.

Power up your pelvic floor

Before you go into a pelvic-floor panic, cross your legs, squeeze and fear that your nether regions are going to fall out, there are ways you can tone up this area.

'Like any muscle, our pelvic-floor muscle gets smaller with age – unless you know how to exercise it and do so regularly,' says Jane. She recommends Kegel (pelvic-floor muscle-training) exercises. 'They're a great way to strengthen the pelvic floor and keep the leaks at bay.'

Follow her five 'firm up' steps:

1. Hold good posture. If you want to work your pelvic floor correctly, you must maintain a tall spine.

2. When seated, make sure you sit on your sit bones with your pelvis straight underneath you.

3. Find your pelvic-floor muscles. First imagine you are stopping passing wind, then stopping a pee. Then think of drawing these two feelings in together and up inside you – the feeling should be between these two points and also between those sit bones you're sitting on – this is where the pelvic floor lies.

4. Breathe! Imagine a cylinder starting underneath your ribcage and finishing at the base of your pelvis, with the spine running down the back of the cylinder, abs around the sides, pelvic floor at the bottom and diaphragm at the top. Breathe in, and the 'cylinder' expands – so the diaphragm, pelvic floor, and deep abdominals widen. Exhale and they contract, and the 'cylinder' gets smaller and tighter. Now lift up your pelvic floor, pulling in your tummy at the same time, so you work the pelvic-floor muscles and improve your deep abdominal strength too.

5. Stretch and relax. The pelvic-floor muscles have to stretch and relax, as well as contract, so always allow time for them to expand, lower and release in between contractions.

The JOY of change

Journalist and broadcaster Caryn Franklin shares her frank account of going through a turbulent menopause and how she came out the other side

'Your boat is on a very choppy sea,' said Maryann knowingly. She is one of the select older and wiser women in my life, who got me through a turbulent period, back there.

I was recounting my story to her with my head in my hands. Life had suddenly become very confusing. Continuing the travel analogy, one minute, I was cruising a marvellously lit highway in a 4x4. The next, without noticing, I had taken a wrong turn, I was bouncing down a dark dirt track in a banger.

'How did I get here?' I kept asking, 'and' (more to the point) 'how can I get out?' I was used to problem-solving and multitasking. Having worked in the fashion industry for more than 30 years, while raising a family, running a business and campaigning for a variety of women's issues, I had not signed up for this

'What if we all knew that menopause could deliver a valuable message of growth and expansion'

EXPERIENCE

chaos. I quickly became anxious about what each new day would hold.

Every woman's experience is different. Menopause is a process of oestrogen and progesterone withdrawal, and will impact on you in a unique way. Everyone I have spoken to laments the taboo nature of talking about what to expect, but perhaps we could all feel less ambivalent about the forthcoming rite of passage, if we knew menopause delivers a mind-blowing midlife recalibration with a valuable message of growth and expansion.

Self-doubt

For me, it started with *Titanic*-sinking feelings, which amplified the tension and discomfort of unresolved problems in my life. I was working hard in a career I loved but one minute I'd be up, the next I'd be wearing a cement straitjacket, hurtling to the bottom of a murky abyss accompanied by the voice of condemnation. 'You really are finished,' it would say.

Then there was the brain fog that convinced me I was going down with early dementia. Industry knowledge evaporated and I found myself unable to remember names, events and dates. My vocabulary shrank too. At home, both daughters would play guessing games to get me to the end of my sentence.

There were minimal physical effects, however. I dutifully utilised insomnia to fit in extra work and I could tolerate the mild heat surges any day, but I know some women are driven to distraction by the intensity of night sweats and daytime hot flushes. I asked my mother and an older girlfriend for insight. The phrases 'Plain sailing' and 'Out the other side in no time,' were bandied about. My GP said I sounded all right to her. ➤

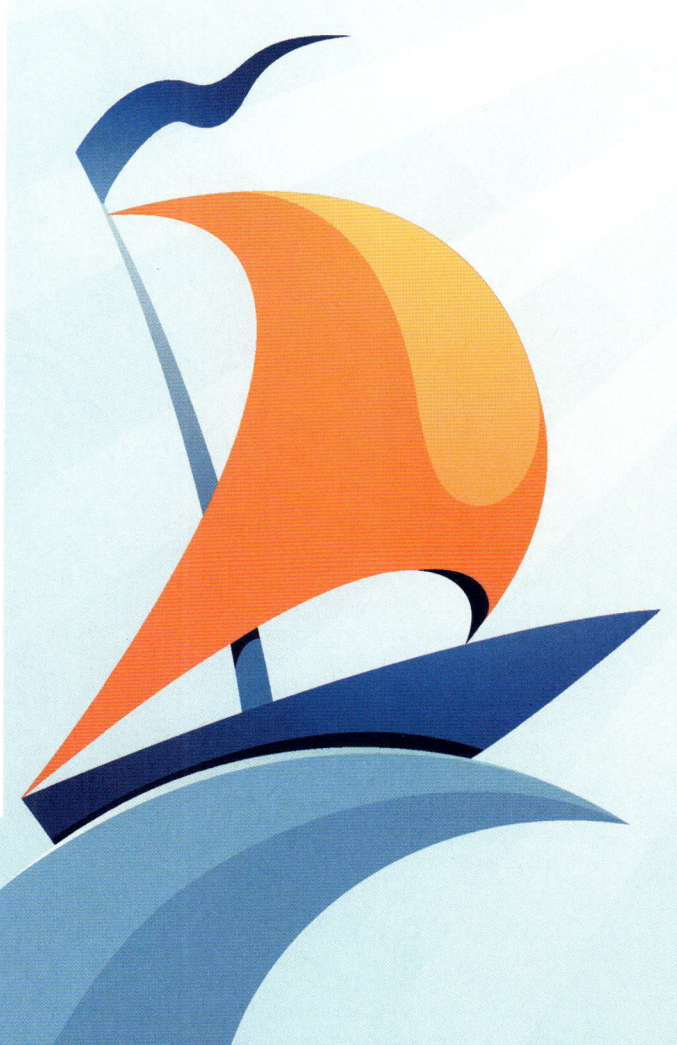

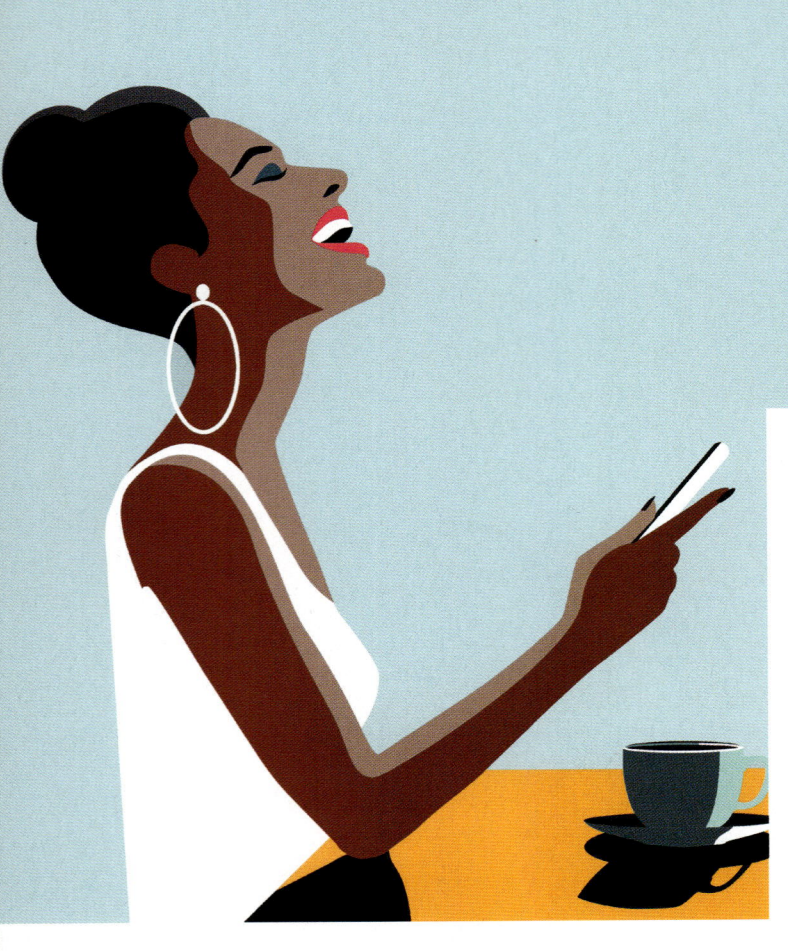

Meanwhile, I was medicating myself with generous amounts of Cabernet Sauvignon each evening. Anaesthetising anxiety this way helped me limp on for a bit longer, clinging to the remnants of my previously ordered existence. Then I made an important decision. I stopped and stood still. 'What do I need to understand?' I asked myself, having read enough to realise that female bodies are powerful, intuitive barometers and mine was trying to tell me something. This is what I learnt…

Cutting myself a break

The voice was right. I was finished. But an ending of the way I had been living would be a very good thing. Since leaving uni, I had put in long hours building a career. As a dedicated parent and partner, I routinely put others first, which meant racing through my life overachieving for others and underprioritising me. Exhausted and running on empty, letting go of my expectations of me would be the first positive move.

In menopause, our body roars. All these years it has put up and shut up, and now will not tolerate abuse or disrespect any longer. This commotion is simply a demand by your newly awake self for quality not quantity, for re-evaluation and rebalancing. Perhaps (when your time comes) you plan to put your hands over your ears? Think again, there is nothing so primal and immediate as your body's hormonal call to action.

I listened. I cut myself a break. As a result, I'm no longer buckling under the stress of numerous projects running concurrently. I've made other changes too. I attend fewer time-wasting meetings, engage in much less unwaged work and collaborate more selectively. I'm thinking about the bigger picture as I celebrate my strengths and focus on the positives, while gracefully accepting my limitations… finally. Now free of hands-on child-wrangling (the final child, birthed at 41, is 20), I'm in an intense relationship with myself. It's a joy, as the voice inside me grows stronger and more enquiring of new perspectives. I have grown my hair and grown out my colour. Shedding old ways and reframing people's perceptions of me, I left the 'People Pleaser' behind. This has been an act of common sense.

'She's let herself go.' A deliberately belittling judgement reveals disapproval of maturing feminine appearance. The assertion that we could try harder to cling on to our youth supports every unrealistic beauty claim for anti-ageing balms and marketing prompt for hair dye. I'm not buying it. In the process of consuming femininity as a set of unrealistic appearance goals, perhaps we have become blind to our internal exquisiteness and it's time to open our eyes. I love fashion and self-styling and I have great fun with my image, but I don't play the game of defining myself as decorative dressing in a man-made world; maybe this has helped me to embrace the privilege of age with its intellectual and experiential gifts. I do believe that if we can stop focusing solely on exteriors and start embracing

> 'Female bodies are powerful, intuitive barometers and mine was trying to tell me something'

> ❝ **I celebrate my strengths, focus on the positives, while gracefully accepting my limitations**

personhood, post-menopause becomes a position of status and composure.

So, for the record… we do not let ourselves go, just the flotsam and jetsam of an earlier existence. The mirror becomes less important with the realisation that age does not equal atrophy and that we are not diminished by the passing of years. Instead we are intensified, our force amplified and our knowledge expanded.

Kindness and tolerance

I now look inwards instead of outwards. Turning up the volume on an inner voice of discernment and overriding the urge to be helpful at the expense of myself, change continues. People who suck the energy out of you can sometimes go undetected when you have energy to spare. But once you decide not to squander your resources, things become clearer. I'm not pretending life miraculously becomes uncomplicated and undemanding – challenges await every age and stage. Women however are great facilitators of others, so in menopause we can and must reclaim our time and assets for ourselves. This is not selfish, this is smart.

The simple truth is that like the adolescent surge of hormonal activity providing an exciting gateway to adult sexuality, menopause (the process in reverse and in withdrawal) enables an equally compelling portal into yet another selfhood. Step towards this doorway with confidence that once out the other side you will be renewed. Prepare yourself mentally and physically beforehand by choosing less stress, more sleep, a healthy diet and supportive friends. Treat yourself with kindness and tolerance as the biochemical make-up of your body rearranges itself. It's an education so expect enlightenment. Post-menopause needs renaming and reclaiming for what it truly is, a magnificent time of curiosity, creativity and rank.

It's not surprising that some societies have been threatened by this natural female evolution. With the introduction of Christianity came the persecution of middle-aged women as witches and heretics. As feminist history explains, older women were simply channelling their menopausal force to intervene in an oppressive culture that undermined female wisdom and equality.

There is no need for any woman to feel ambivalent, even fearful, of ageing. In fact with the right physical, emotional and mental health supports we can thrive. Hearing other women's stories at the time I was at my worst, helped me and I wish the same for you. Now, having roused the ancient mystic and tribal elder in me, I am on the journey towards cronehood and I love it.

✦ **Caryn has contributed to FASHION – A Definitive Visual Guide** (£21, Dorling Kindersley)

> **Step towards this doorway with confidence that once out the other side you will be renewed**

'Woman are great facilitators of others, so in menopause we can and must reclaim our time and assets for ourselves'

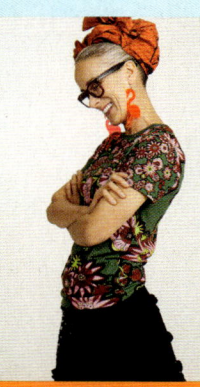

Styling it out

Fashion commentator and stylist, Caryn is perhaps best known for presenting BBC's *The Clothes Show* but has always been interested in the politics of image and self-esteem. Now 61, and with an MSc in Applied Psychology in Selfhood, Objectification, Inclusivity and Gender Bias, Caryn continues to write, present and teach while advising industry on the benefits of diverse perspectives. She's currently a visiting professor of diverse selfhood at Kingston School of Art.

Eat yourself happy & healthy

What we eat in menopause can influence how we feel. In *Superfoods to Superhealth,* Dr Johanna Ward offers dietary advice and inspiring recipes

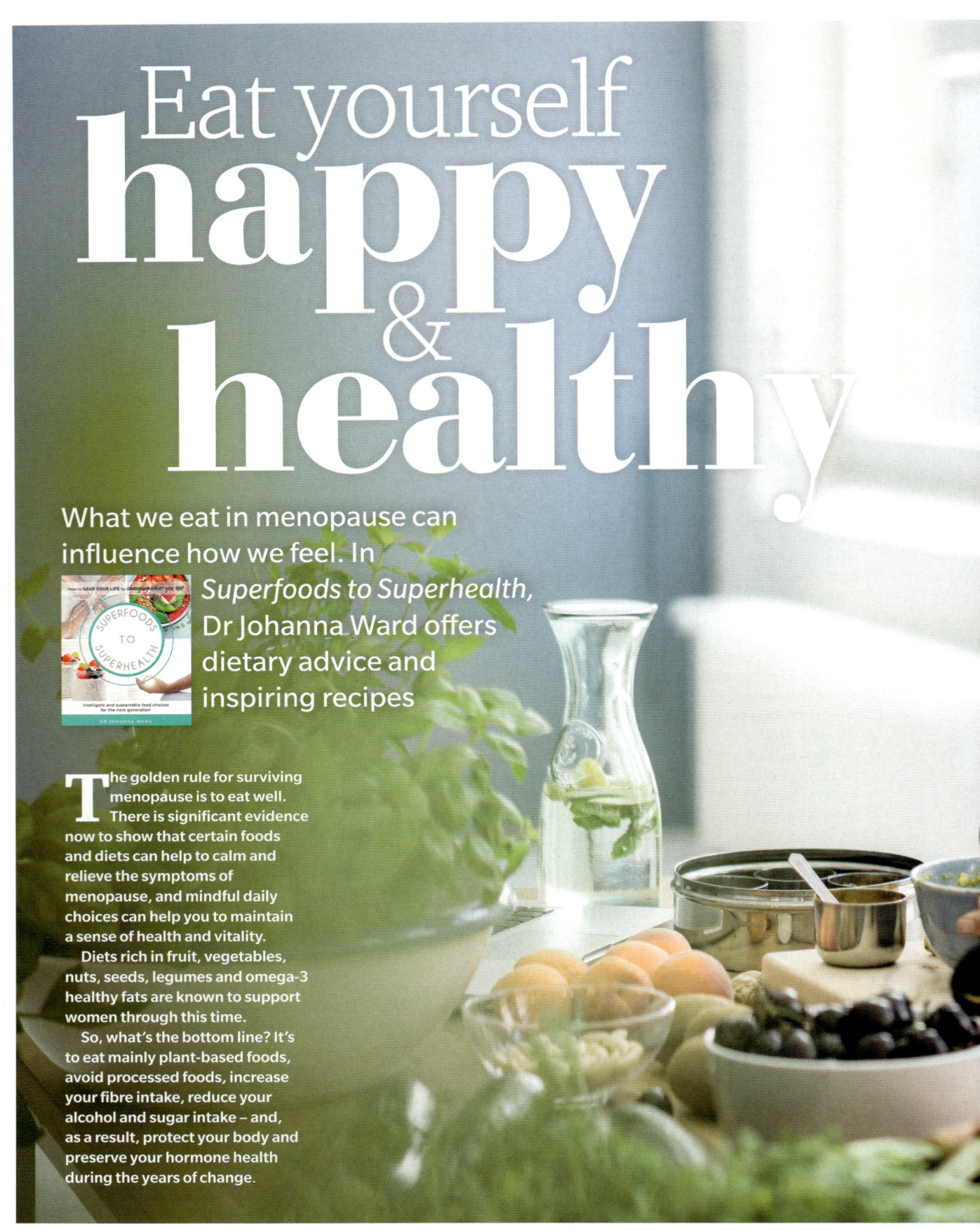

The golden rule for surviving menopause is to eat well. There is significant evidence now to show that certain foods and diets can help to calm and relieve the symptoms of menopause, and mindful daily choices can help you to maintain a sense of health and vitality.

Diets rich in fruit, vegetables, nuts, seeds, legumes and omega-3 healthy fats are known to support women through this time.

So, what's the bottom line? It's to eat mainly plant-based foods, avoid processed foods, increase your fibre intake, reduce your alcohol and sugar intake – and, as a result, protect your body and preserve your hormone health during the years of change.

NUTRITION

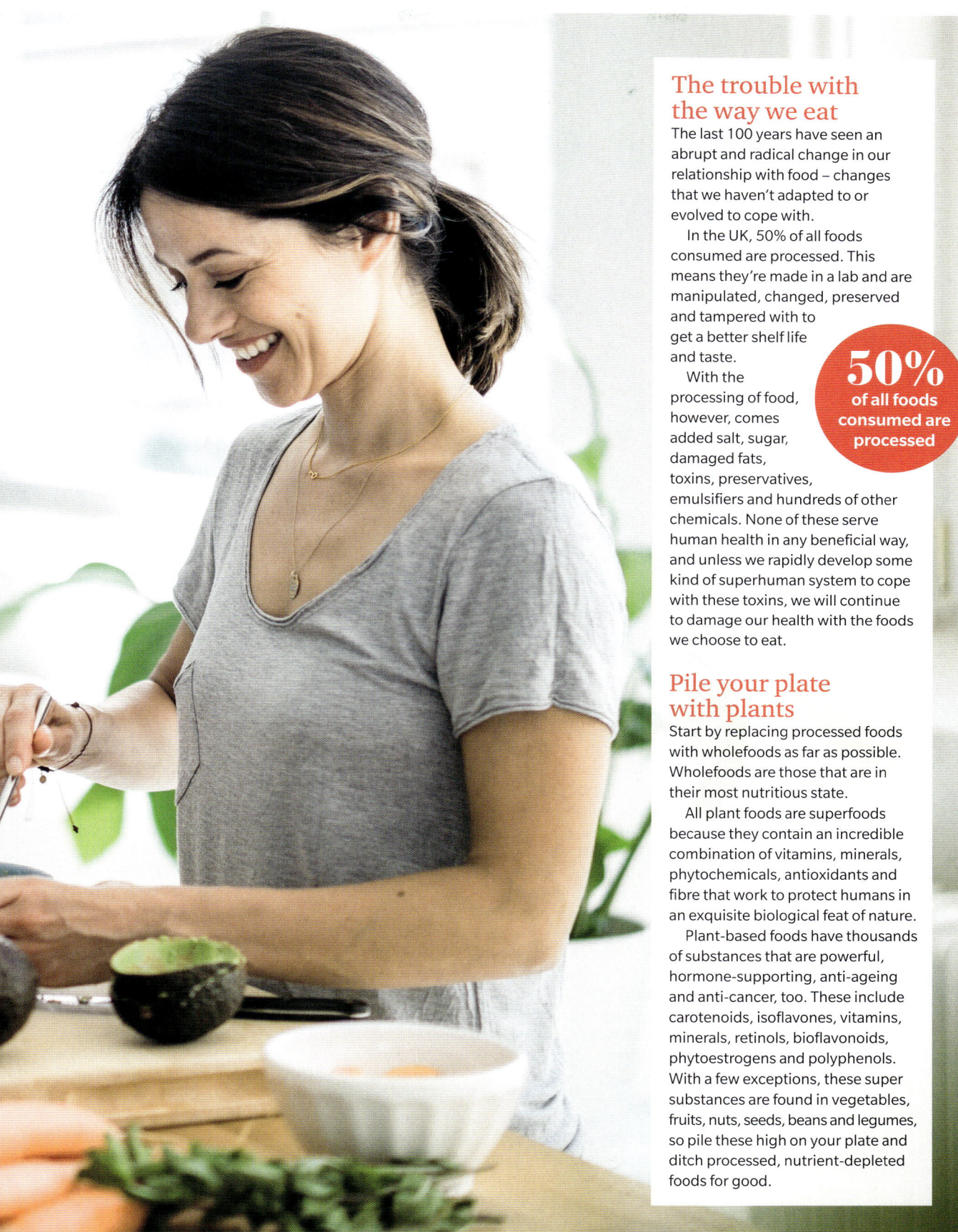

The trouble with the way we eat

The last 100 years have seen an abrupt and radical change in our relationship with food – changes that we haven't adapted to or evolved to cope with.

In the UK, 50% of all foods consumed are processed. This means they're made in a lab and are manipulated, changed, preserved and tampered with to get a better shelf life and taste.

With the processing of food, however, comes added salt, sugar, damaged fats, toxins, preservatives, emulsifiers and hundreds of other chemicals. None of these serve human health in any beneficial way, and unless we rapidly develop some kind of superhuman system to cope with these toxins, we will continue to damage our health with the foods we choose to eat.

50% of all foods consumed are processed

Pile your plate with plants

Start by replacing processed foods with wholefoods as far as possible. Wholefoods are those that are in their most nutritious state.

All plant foods are superfoods because they contain an incredible combination of vitamins, minerals, phytochemicals, antioxidants and fibre that work to protect humans in an exquisite biological feat of nature.

Plant-based foods have thousands of substances that are powerful, hormone-supporting, anti-ageing and anti-cancer, too. These include carotenoids, isoflavones, vitamins, minerals, retinols, bioflavonoids, phytoestrogens and polyphenols. With a few exceptions, these super substances are found in vegetables, fruits, nuts, seeds, beans and legumes, so pile these high on your plate and ditch processed, nutrient-depleted foods for good.

The Smart Woman's Guide to the Menopause

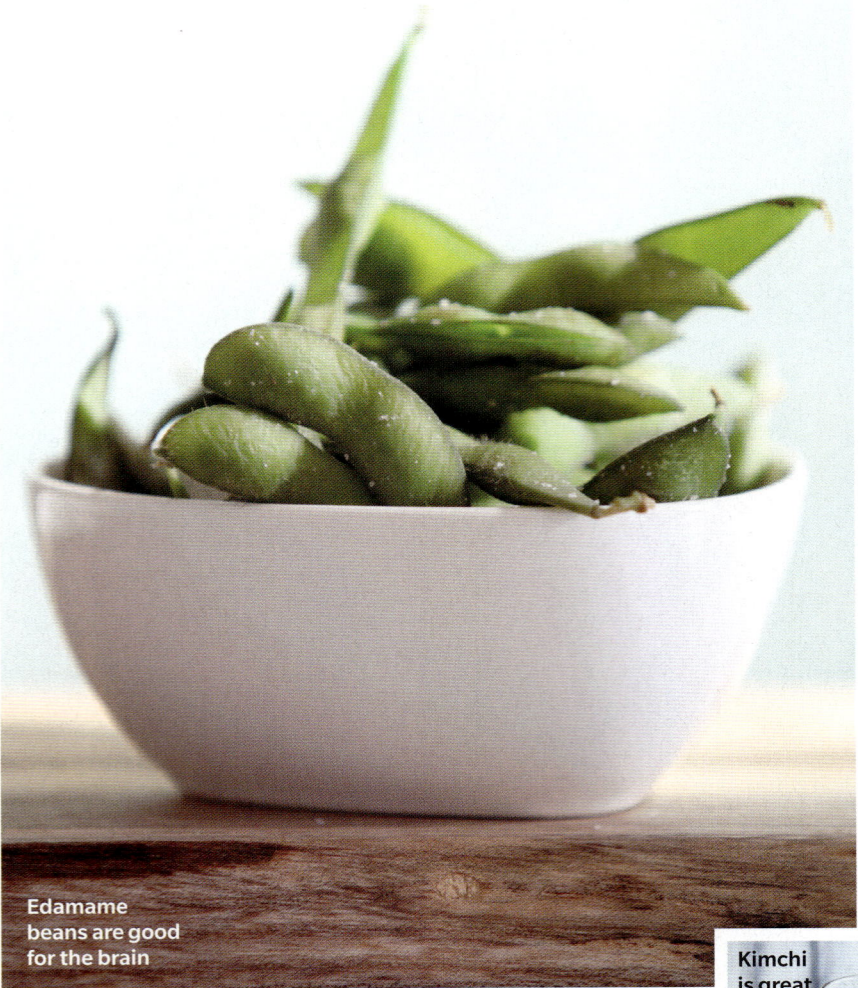
Edamame beans are good for the brain

Why hormones matter

1 The average age of menopause in the UK is 51. This means that many women will live their last 30 or more years without oestrogen, progesterone and testosterone – all important anabolic hormones.

2 Hormones are powerful chemical communicators and signal some of the most important life events, such as birth, growth, puberty and ageing. As a society, we have historically failed to understand the importance of female hormone health. Women who are low, exhausted or prone to mood swings have been labelled 'hard work' or even 'crazy'! But the importance of hormone health cannot be overestimated.

3 Hormones affect everything from brain function and heart health to mood and libido, and when they are crashing, women can feel overwhelmed and out of control. Balancing hormones is critical to bringing a sense of calm, empowerment and wellbeing to women in menopause. Knowing how to support your hormones through diet and lifestyle can be life-changing.

AN EXTRA BOOST
Improve your mind and body with:
- Valerian root or melatonin supplements for insomnia.
- Black cohosh, red clover and sage for hot flushes.
- Red clover and sage for night sweats.
- Ginkgo biloba to improve blood flow and brain health.
- Omega-3 to protect brain function.
- B6 for serotonin production.
- D3 for immunity and bone support.
- Marine collagen for joint, bone, skin and hair support.
- Johanna's own supplement, ZENii Rebalance – a blend of soya isoflavones, red clover, kelp, pfaffia, wild yam and sage leaf with ginsneg, zinc and vitamin B6 – is £35 for 60 capsules (zenii.co.uk).

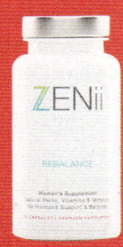

Care for your gut

We have over 100 trillion microbes inside us. These essential microbes help guide, process, feed and even 'hijack' our own genetic material.

As we age, a lot of these beneficial bacteria deplete in number, impacting everything from our immunity to our ability to create hormones. That's why it's so important to nurture our gut health and to try and repopulate our microbiome with healthy food and lifestyle choices.

The profound connection between the gut and our immune and neurochemical systems is finally being recognised, and we are starting to understand the missing pieces of the puzzle that underpins health. The 'crosstalk' between all of our systems is huge. Gut microbiota help to regulate everything from our immunity and libido to brain health and hormone health.

Eating in a way that supports our gut is especially important during menopause, with the emphasis on prebiotic, probiotic and fibre-rich foods. A plant-based diet will contain these three gut-boosting properties. Add in some fermented foods, like kimchi, miso, tempeh and kombucha, and you will be helping to feed and boost your microbial population.

Exposure to certain medicines, chemicals and foods can adversely affect your intestinal microbes. Medicines like antibiotics, the contraceptive pill, NSAIDs (for example, ibuprofen, neurofen) and acid blockers like omeprazole all deplete good bacteria. Antibiotics kill good and bad bacteria, so they decimate the general bacterial population, and it can take months to years to regain a healthy balance. Alcohol, chronic stress and exposure to pesticides can all harm our beneficial bacteria, so filter your water, reduce your alcohol intake and eat organic to improve your gut's functionality.

Kimchi is great for gut health

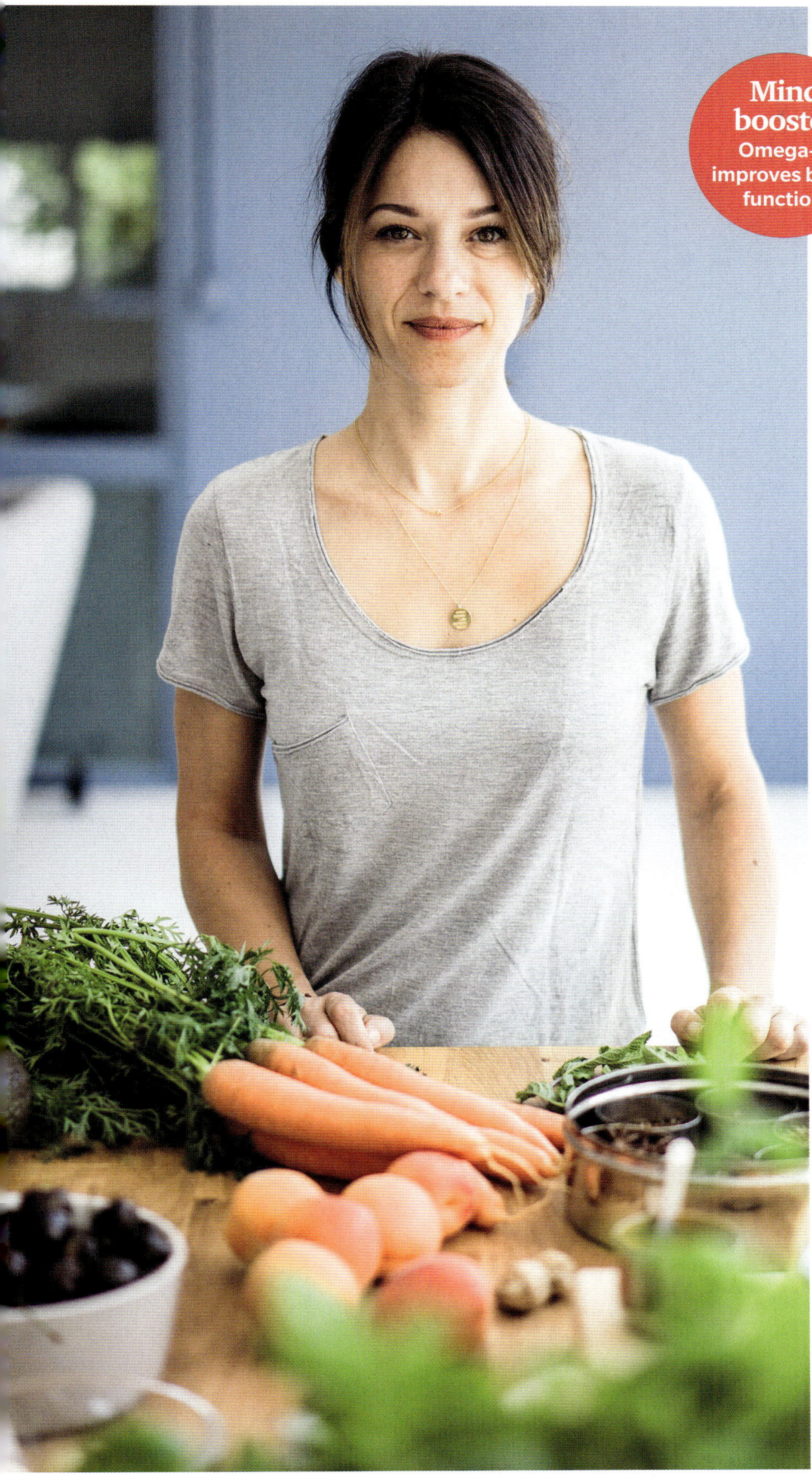

NUTRITION

Feed your brain

Mind booster
Omega-3 improves brain function

During menopause, many women experience brain fog, poor memory, low mood and fatigue. Cutting out processed foods, reducing sugar and eating low-GI foods can have profound benefits, as can increasing your intake of omega-3, antioxidants, phytonutrients, vitamins B, C, D and E, and good-quality protein.

Numerous studies prove that a higher omega-3 intake reduces the incidence of brain disorders, such as Alzheimer's and vascular dementia. Deficiencies in DHA, which comprises 90% of the brain's omega-3 fatty acids, have been linked to poor memory, attention span and learning.

Most of the body's serotonin – the happy hormone – is made in the gut and is produced more abundantly when we eat tryptophan. Chia seeds are a wonderful source, as are edamame beans, prunes, spirulina and natural yogurt.

Turn the page for recipes ➤

Food for thought
Science behind the facts...

✦ In a study of over 17,000 menopausal women, those eating more unprocessed soy products, veg, fruit and fibre experienced a 19% reduction in hot flushes.

✦ Another study showed that omega-3 supplements decreased the frequency of hot flushes and the severity of night sweats.

✦ An ongoing study published in the *British Medical Journal* showed that three servings a day of whole grains like quinoa, brown rice and kamut wheat reduced the incidence of heart disease, cancer and premature death in menopausal women.

✦ High circulating blood sugars have been associated with increased incidence of hot flushes, weight gain and poor sleep. Opting for a low-GI diet is the best option.

✦ Alcohol and caffeine are known to trigger hot flushes and should be avoided if possible.

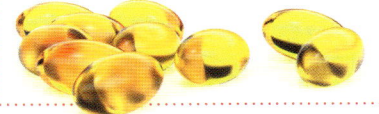

The Smart Woman's Guide to the Menopause

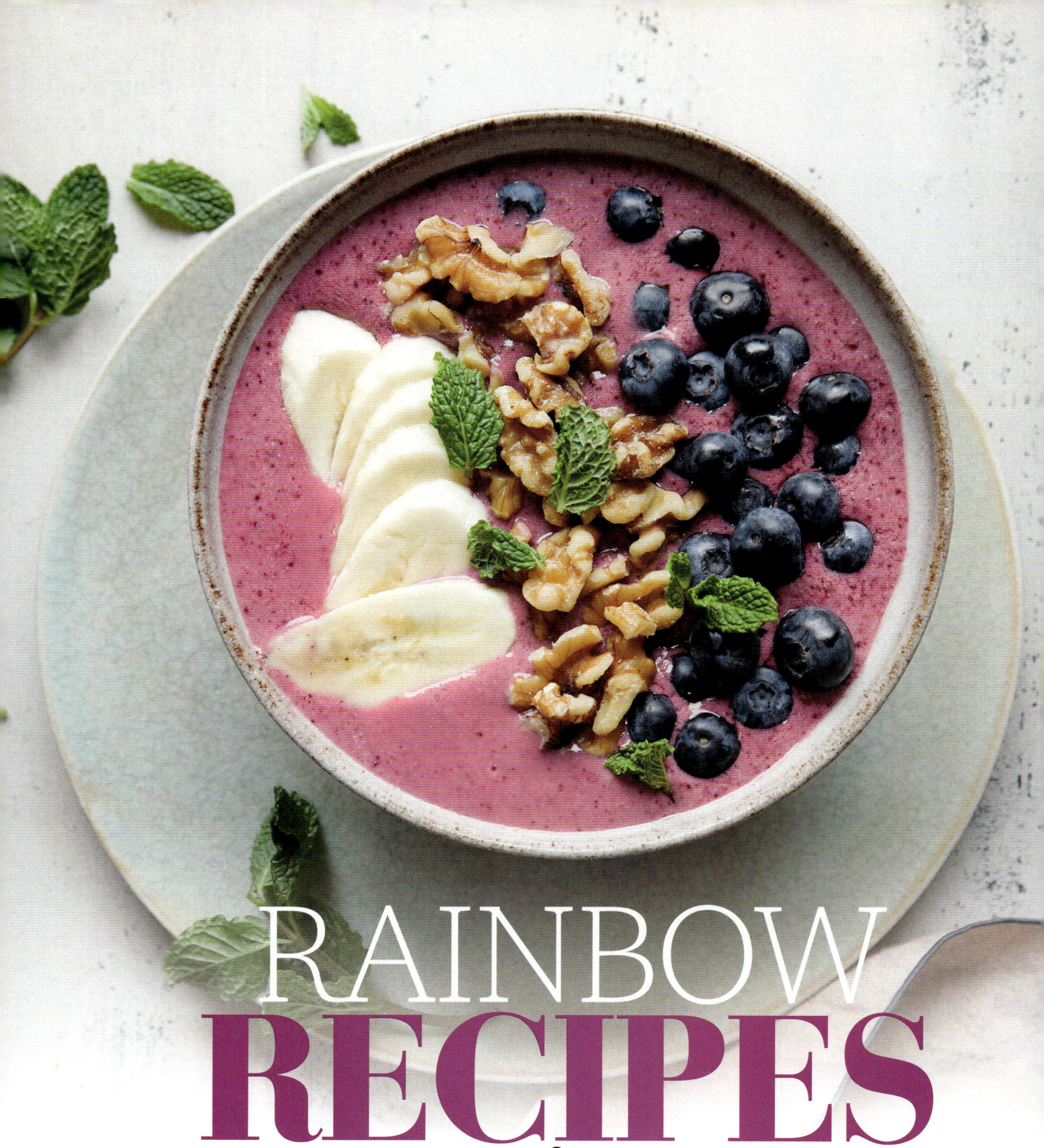

RAINBOW RECIPES to revive you

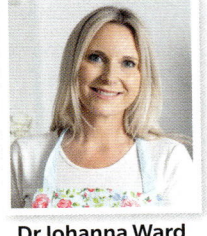
Dr Johanna Ward

Dr Johanna Ward and plant-based chef Charlotte Kjaer bring you five delicious dishes packed with the nutrients you need for midlife...

RECIPES

'Superbug' smoothie

'Kefir is a fermented food rich in probiotics. Coconut kefir is a wonderful, dairy-free way of repopulating the gut with beneficial bacteria that can be added to any smoothie for extra gut-health benefits,' says Johanna. 'I like to add probiotics, prebiotics and spirulina powders as well. Your gut has more bugs in it than humans have ever populated this planet – so it pays to look after them.'

Serves 2 Gluten-free
- 250ml coconut water
- 1 cup frozen mixed berries
- 1 banana, sliced, reserving a few slices
- 1 tsp flaxseed
- ½ lemon, squeezed
- coconut kefir

Topping:
- handful of blueberries
- handful walnuts
- few mint leaves
- probiotic, acai and chlorella powders (optional)

Blend all the ingredients in a jug blender, then serve topped with reserved banana, blueberries, walnuts, mint leaves and powders, if using.

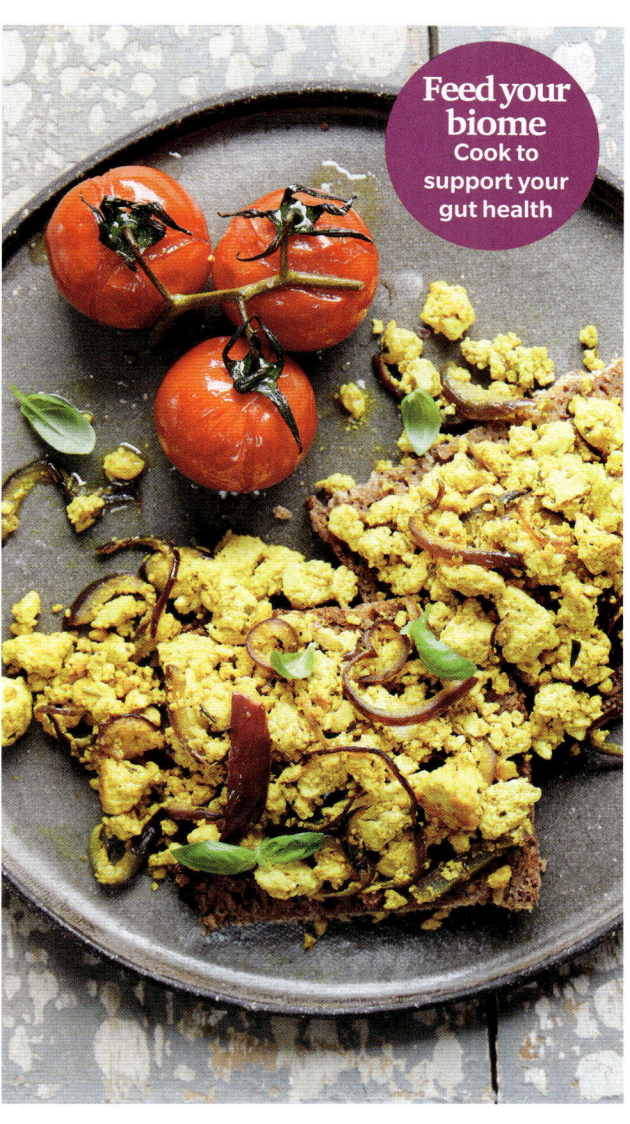

Feed your biome Cook to support your gut health

Scrambled tofu, red onion and roast tomato breakfast

Serves 4
Gluten-free, nut-free
- 8 tomatoes on the vine
- 300g organic tofu
- 1 tsp turmeric
- 1 tsp black pepper
- 1 tsp oregano or mixed herbs
- 1 red onion
- coconut oil
- handful of fresh basil

1. Heat the oven to 180C/Gas 4. Place the vine tomatoes onto a baking tray, drizzle with olive oil, season and roast for 7-10 minutes until soft.
2. Crumble the tofu into small pieces in a mixing bowl. Add the turmeric, black pepper, herbs and salt and mix well.
3. Slice the onion and fry in coconut oil until soft and translucent, add the tofu and fry until slightly crisp and golden brown, around 3-5 minutes. Serve on rye bread with the vine tomatoes and freshly torn basil.

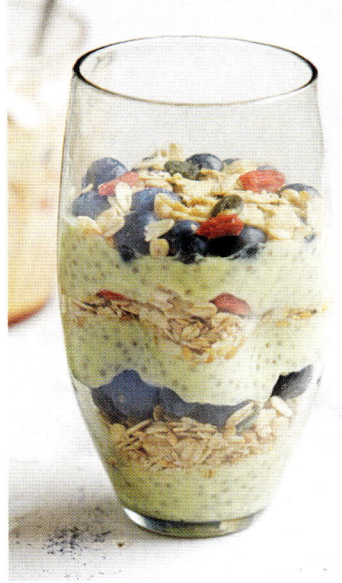

Creamy coconut mango chia pudding with blueberries and toasted coconut chips

'Chia seeds are one of my favourite superfoods,' says Johanna. 'They have been eaten for centuries in South America and are now becoming popular here in the UK. Chias have so much to offer nutritionally. They're rich in tryptophan – an essential amino acid that's a precursor to serotonin and melatonin. Both help us to feel happy, calm and content. Chias are also high in ALA omega-3 fatty acids, fibre, calcium, zinc and phosphorous.'

Serves 4-6
Gluten-free, nut-free
- 1 ripe mango
- 3tbsp chia seeds
- 400ml tin coconut milk
- 1 lime, juice and zest
- 1tbsp vanilla or vanilla pod
- blueberries, coconut chips and a few dried cranberries, to serve

1. Peel and dice the mango, then place in a jug blender with the lime juice and zest and blend until smooth and creamy.
2. Add the coconut milk to the mango and vanilla and blend together.
3. Place the mixture in a bowl, add the chia seeds and mix well.
4. Cover and refrigerate for around 30mins to set. If the mixture feels too loose, add 1 tbsp more of chia and leave it to thicken.
5. Serve the chia mixture in glasses or bowls, layered with coconut chips, blueberries and cranberries, finishing with a layer of fruit and coconut.

The Smart Woman's Guide to the Menopause

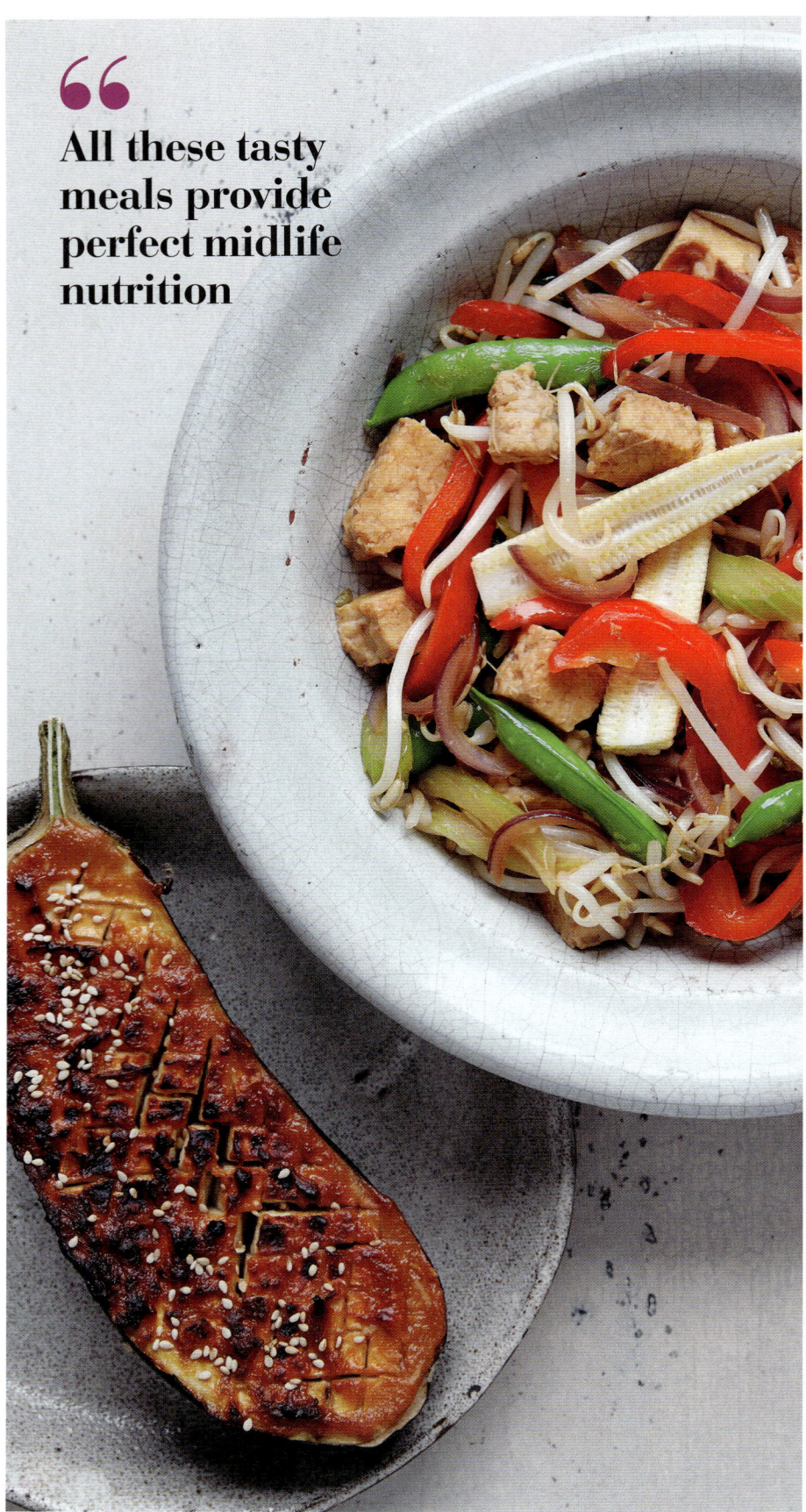

> "All these tasty meals provide perfect midlife nutrition"

Miso roast aubergine with tempeh and stir-fry vegetables

Serves 2 Gluten-free, nut-free
- 1 pack (300g) tempeh
- coconut oil

Tempeh marinade:
- 2 tbsp tamari soy sauce
- 1 tbsp rice wine vinegar
- 3 garlic cloves, crushed
- 1 inch ginger, grated

Aubergine:
- 1 aubergine
- 2 tbsp miso paste
- 1 garlic clove, crushed
- 1 tsp sesame seeds
- 1 tsp nigella seeds

Stir-fry vegetables:
- 6 baby corn, sliced
- 1 red pepper, sliced
- 100g mangetout
- 100g bean sprouts
- 1 red onion, sliced
- 1 celery stalk, chopped

1 Preheat the oven to 180C/Gas 4. Make the tempeh marinade by putting all the ingredients into a bowl and mixing well. Cut the tempeh into 1cm cubes and add to the marinade.

2 Cut the aubergine lengthways down the centre and score the flesh diagonally, being careful not to cut all the way through. Place the miso, garlic and 1 tbsp water into a bowl and whisk until combined. Brush over the miso marinade and place on a baking tray, cover lightly with foil and roast for 15 minutes until the aubergine is soft. Remove the foil, sprinkle with the seeds and roast for 5 more minutes to caramelise.

3 Meanwhile, heat 2 tbsp coconut oil in a large frying pan, remove the tempeh from the marinade and fry for 5 minutes. Add the stir-fry vegetables to the pan with the tempeh and fry for 5 minutes more until softened but still crisp. Pour over the remaining marinade and mix well. Serve with the roasted aubergine in its skin.

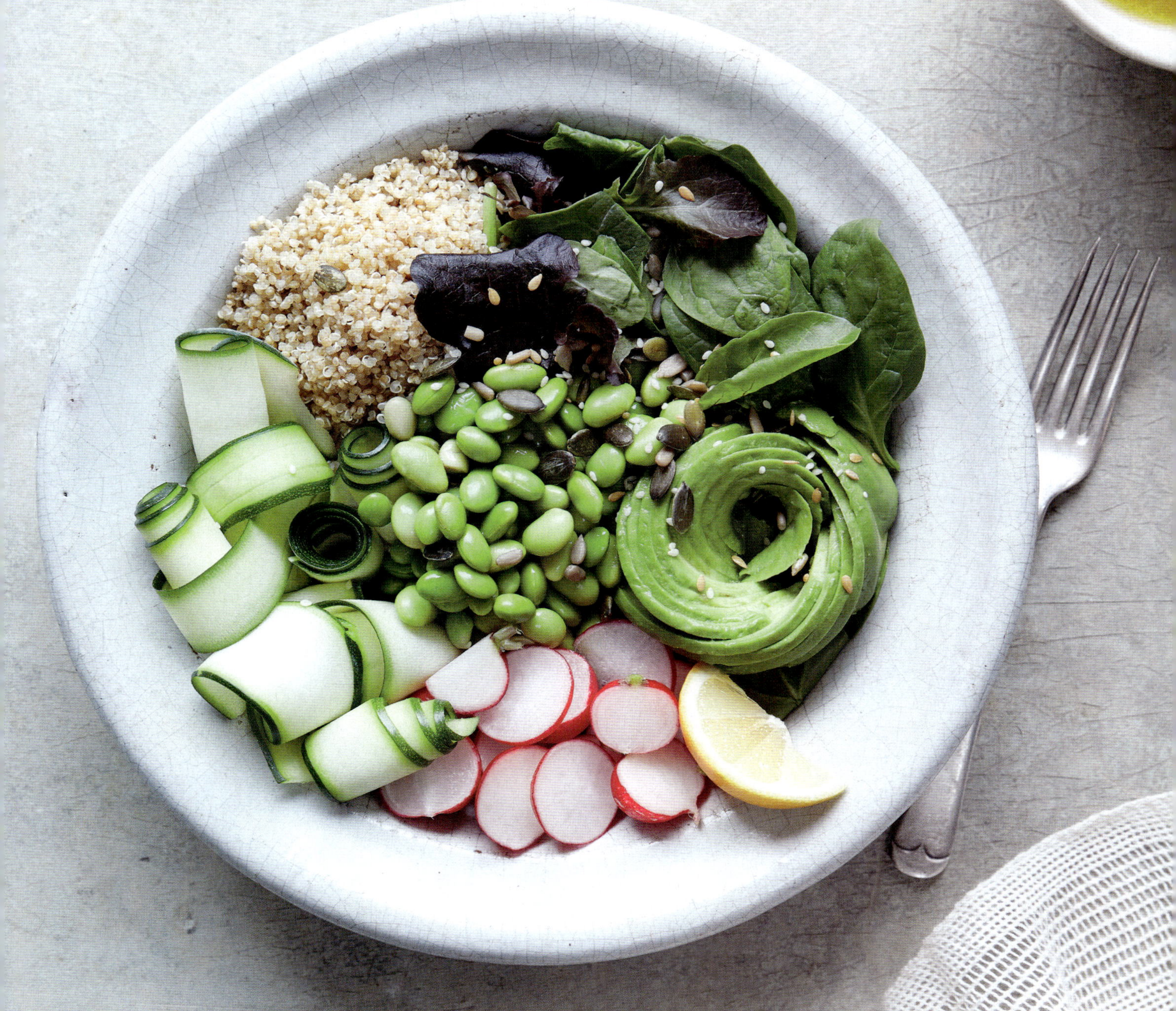

RECIPES

Summer Buddha bowl of edamame, courgette and avocado with lemon vinaigrette

'Edamame beans are young soy beans that have been harvested early. They are a complete protein and a highly nutritious plant-based food. Loaded with vitamins and minerals and high in polyunsaturated ALA fats, edamame beans are also high in folate, which reduces homocysteine levels and genistein, the predominant isoflavone in soy which is known to inhibit the growth of cancer cells. They are soft beans, unlike the mature beans used to make soy milk and tofu.'

Serves 2 Gluten-free, nut-free
- 100g quinoa
- ½ courgette
- 50g peas
- 75g edamame beans
- 1 avocado, peeled and sliced
- handful of small radish, sliced
- handful of salad leaves

Dressing:
- 1 lemon, juiced, plus wedges
- 2 tbsp olive oil
- 1 tsp Dijon mustard
- 1 garlic clove, crushed

1. Cook the quinoa according to the packet instructions.
2. Use a vegetable peeler to cut thin curls of the courgette.
3. Defrost the peas in warm water for a few minutes, then drain and combine with the beans. Meanwhile, make the dressing by whisking the ingredients in a bowl.
4. To serve, place the quinoa and leaves in shallow bowls, add the vegetables, pour over the dressing and garnish with lemon wedges.

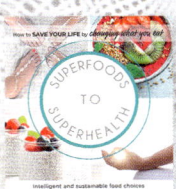

Superfoods to Superhealth by Dr Johanna Ward, £27, from Amazon

The Smart Woman's Guide to the Menopause

Asparagus, bean, mushroom and miso salad

Three plant-based nutrients provide a three-way attack on hot flushes.

Serves 4
Prep: 10 mins
Cook: 10 mins

- 200g asparagus, trimmed
- 200g green beans, trimmed and halved
- 200g Tenderstem broccoli
- 1 tbsp olive oil
- 8 shiitake mushrooms
- 1 red onion, sliced
- 2 cloves garlic, crushed
- 2 Little Gem lettuces
- 5g pack crispy seaweed (such as Itsu Crispy Seaweed Thins from Waitrose)
- 1 tbsp tahini
- 2 tbsp sweet white miso paste
- 2 tbsp lemon juice
- 1 tsp tamari or soy sauce

1. Boil asparagus, beans and broccoli in for 3 mins until just tender. Drain.
2. Heat oil in a frying pan, add mushrooms, red onion and garlic and cook for 5 mins to soften, then add 2tbsp water and cook for a further 2 mins.
3. Divide Little Gem leaves between four plates. Combine the vegetables, pile on top and scatter over]crispy seaweed.
4. Make a dressing: mix tahini, miso paste, lemon juice and tamari or soy sauce together. Drizzle over salad to serve.

Per serving: 134 cals, 6g fat (1g sat fat), 8g carbs

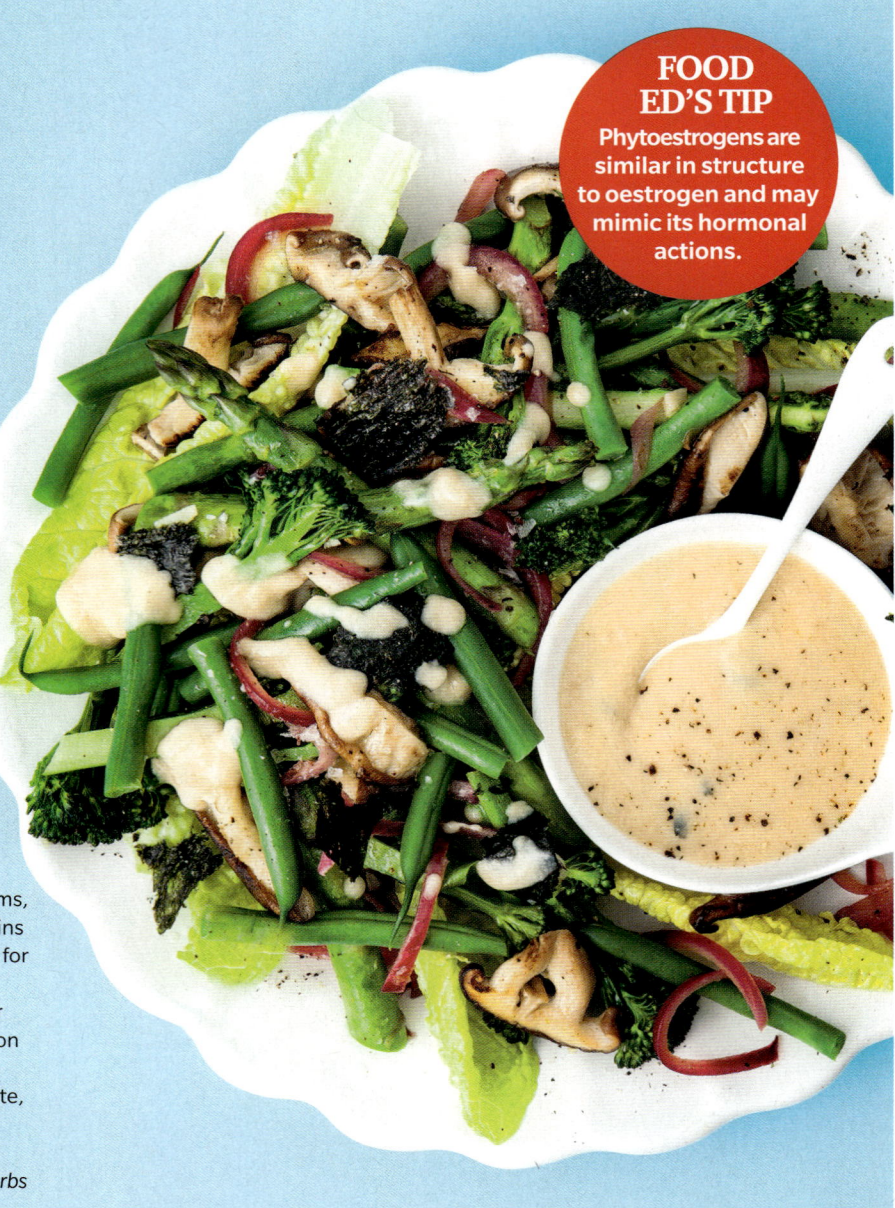

FOOD ED'S TIP
Phytoestrogens are similar in structure to oestrogen and may mimic its hormonal actions.

EAT TO BEAT HOT FLUSHES

These dishes are rich in phytoestrogens that help the body to manage menopausal symptoms

Nutrition

Teriyaki salmon with edamame beans

Salmon is rich in omega-3, which is thought to help ease the symptoms of depression associated with menopause, as well as hot flushes.

Serves 4
Prep: 5 mins
Cook: 15 mins

- 4 x 125g salmon fillets
- 4tbsp teriyaki sauce
- 200g fresh or frozen edamame beans (without pods)
- 4 egg noodle nests
- 1 bunch of spring onions, dark ends shredded, the rest sliced

1. Put the salmon fillets into a shallow dish and pour over the teriyaki sauce. Heat a griddle pan and pan-fry the salmon with the sauce for 10 mins, turning once.
2. Microwave frozen edamame beans for 2-3 mins (1-2 mins if fresh). Cook noodles in boiling salted water for 4 mins, then drain. Flash-fry spring onion until tender.
3. Serve salmon on a bed of edamame and spring onions, drizzled with teriyaki sauce, with noodles on the side.

Per serving: 532 cals, 21g fat (4g sat fat), 47g carbs

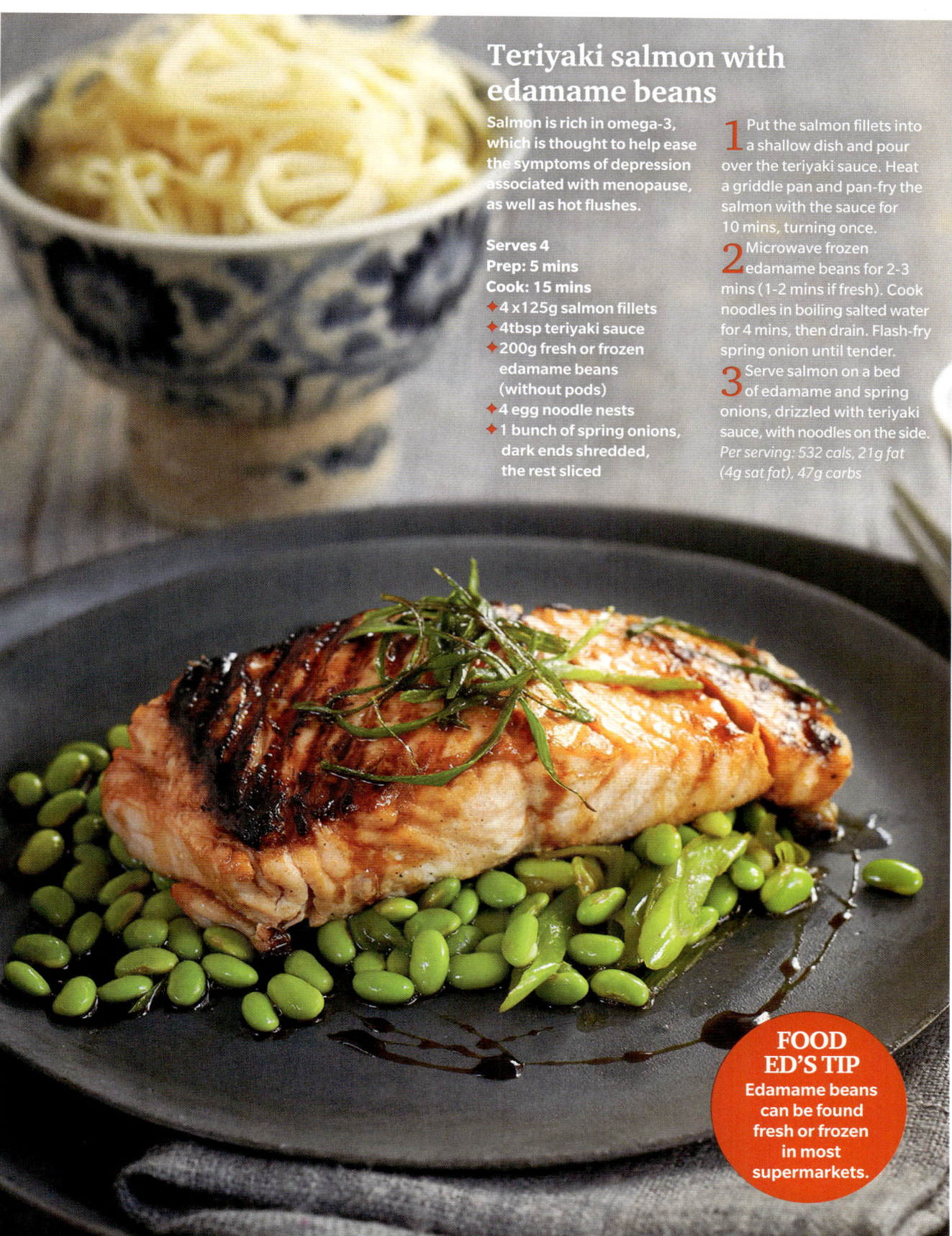

FOOD ED'S TIP
Edamame beans can be found fresh or frozen in most supermarkets.

The Smart Woman's Guide to the Menopause

Granola with mango and yogurt

This can be served either as a healthy dessert or a filling breakfast. Oats, flax and soy yogurt are the sources of phytoestrogens here, and the nuts provide omega-3.

Serves 2, plus extra granola
Prep: 10 mins
Cook: 25 mins

- 2tbsp coconut oil
- 125ml maple syrup
- 1tsp vanilla extract
- 250g jumbo oats
- 100g sunflower seeds
- 100g sesame seeds
- 30g flax seeds
- 100g each of pecans and almonds, chopped
- 60g coconut flakes
- 250g soy yogurt
- 1 mango, peeled, stoned and diced
- Seeds of 1 passion fruit

1. Preheat the oven to 140C/Gas 3. Gently heat the coconut oil, maple syrup and vanilla in a pan together until melted, then stir well.
2. Line 2 baking trays with baking paper. Sprinkle half of the oats, sunflower, sesame and flax seeds, pecans and almonds over each tray.
3. Drizzle each with the maple syrup mixture and bake for 15 mins, then stir and cook for a further 5-10 mins.
4. Once cool, transfer the granola mix to a large bowl and stir in the coconut flakes.
5. Divide the soy yogurt between two bowls and top each with 60g granola and half the mango and scooped-out passion fruit seeds.

Per serving: 423 cals, 24g fat (6g sat fat), 32g carbs

FOOD ED'S TIP
For maximum benefit at breakfast, serve the extra granola with soy milk.

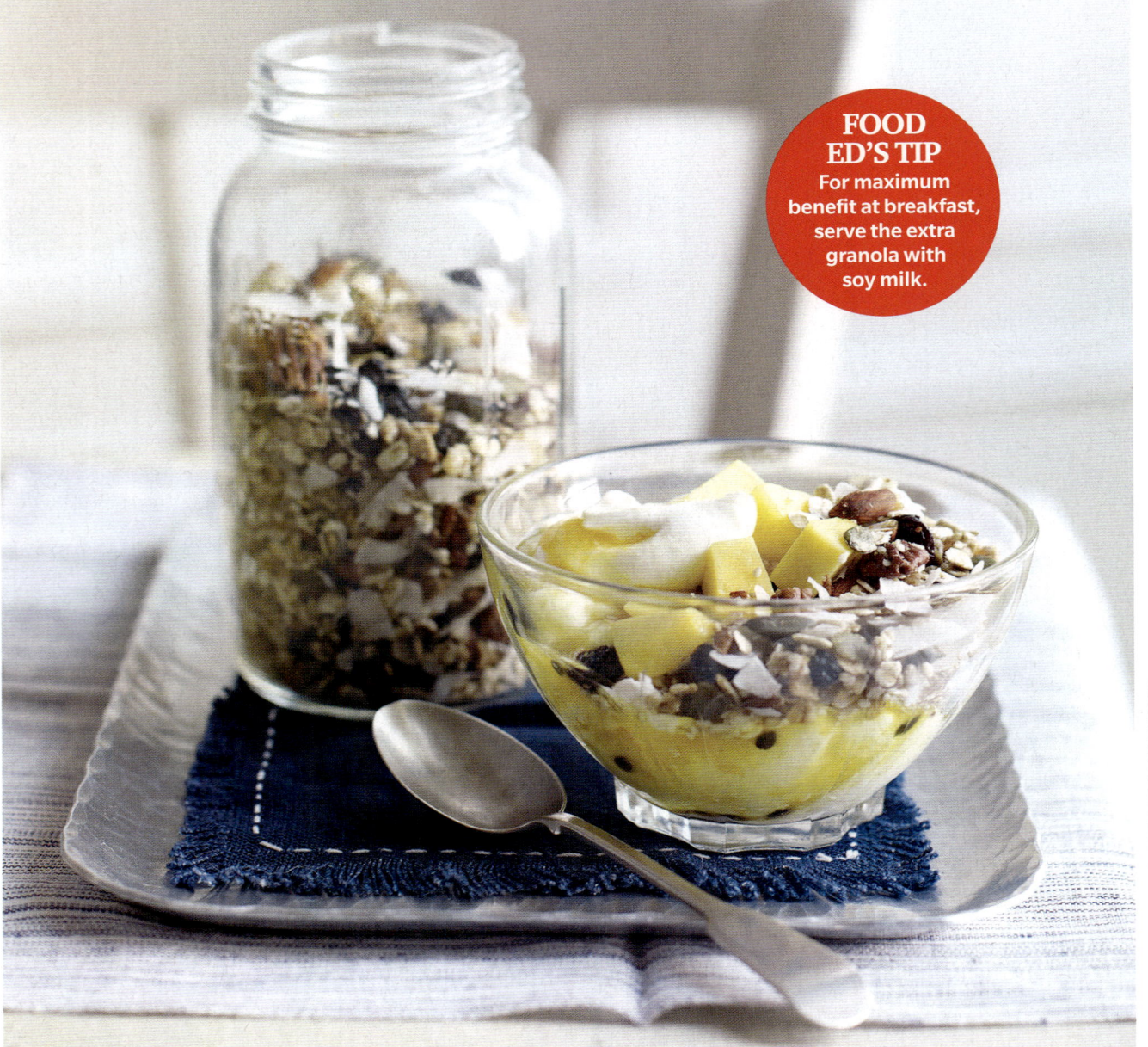

NUTRITION

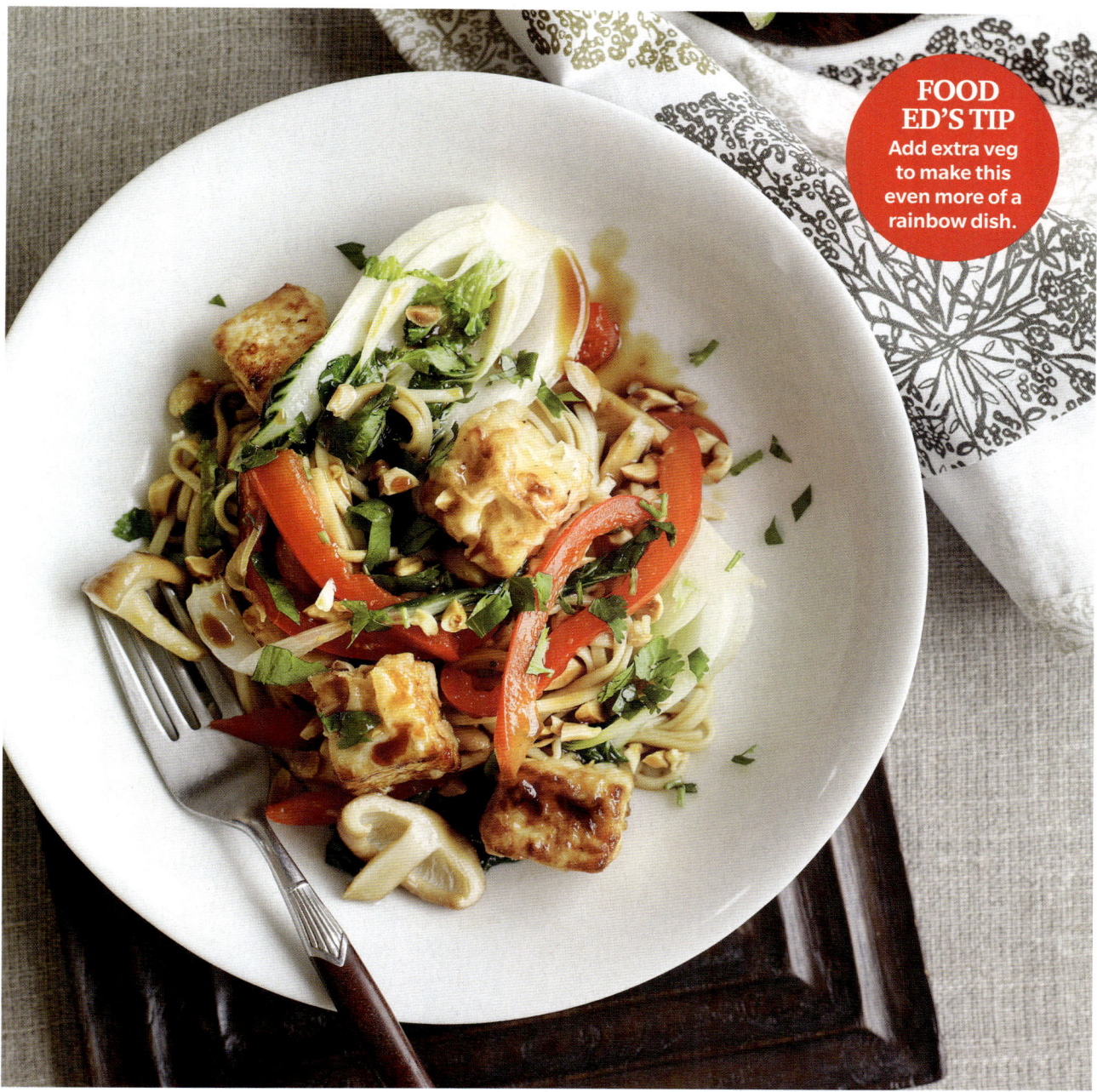

FOOD ED'S TIP
Add extra veg to make this even more of a rainbow dish.

Tofu and peanut stir-fry with ramen noodles

This speedy dish is packed with goodness and would make a substantial lunch or light supper.

Serves 4
Prep: 10 mins
Cook: 10 mins

- 5tbsp sunflower oil
- 350g firm silken tofu, cut into chunks
- 3tbsp seasoned plain flour
- 1 onion, sliced
- 1 red pepper, sliced
- 4tbsp teriyaki sauce
- 150g shiitake mushrooms, sliced
- 8 baby pak choi, halved lengthways
- 250g ramen noodles, cooked and tossed in a little oil
- Juice of 2 limes, plus lime wedges to garnish, if liked
- Coriander and toasted peanuts, to garnish

1. Heat 3tbsp of the oil in a frying pan until it starts to shimmer. Meanwhile, toss tofu in the seasoned flour, then fry in the tofu in batches until golden and crisp on the outside. Drain on kitchen paper and set aside.

2. Heat a wok and add the remaining oil. When it's smoking hot, add the onion, then the pepper, teriyaki sauce and mushrooms. Cook, tossing the veg around often, for a few mins, then add the pak choi, noodles, tofu and lime juice.

3. Serve in bowls, sprinkled with the coriander and peanuts, with extra lime wedges on the side if you like.

Per serving: 540 cals, 21g fat (3g sat fat), 67g carbs

The Smart Woman's Guide to the Menopause

Feed the hormone rollercoaster

Fill your shopping basket with these foods to give your body an easier ride

Whatever stage of the menopause you're going through, it's likely your hormones could be making things a little tricky. 'All women will have a different experience of the perimenopause and the menopause,' explains menopause specialist Kathy Abernethy. 'While there's no such thing as an ideal menopause diet, there's no doubt that some foods will become particularly relevant at this time of life.' Here's what to eat to help create calm…

NUTRITION

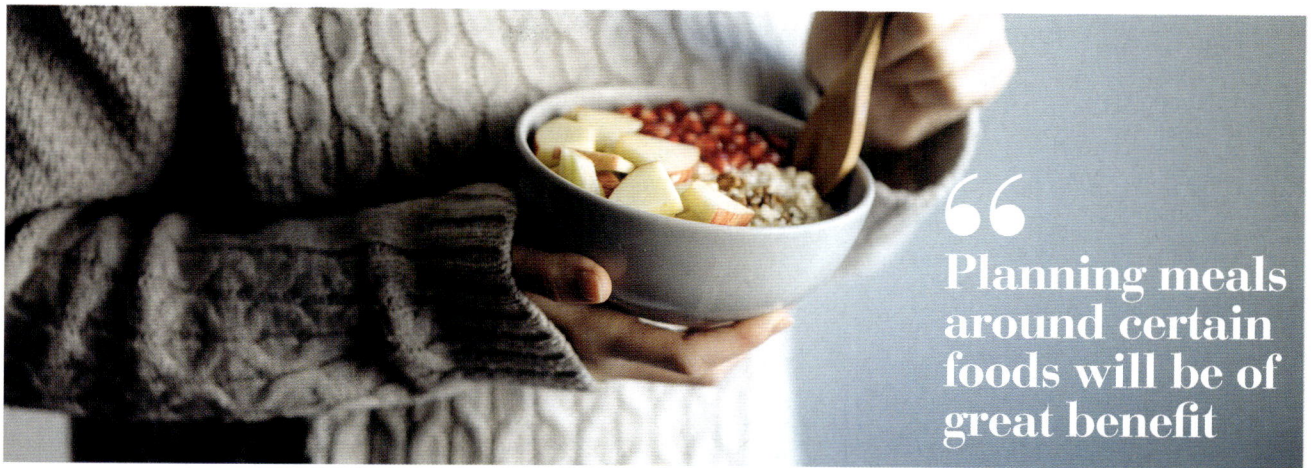

> "Planning meals around certain foods will be of great benefit"

■ SHATAVARI
An Ayurvedic herb that helps stabilise hormones. 'Taken regularly, it can be supportive for those struggling with hot flushes, vaginal dryness, low libido and low mood,' says medical herbalist Katie Pande. Shatavari can be taken in capsule form and also drunk in a tea. **Try Pukka Wholistic Shatavari (£16.95 for 30 capsules, ocado.com).**

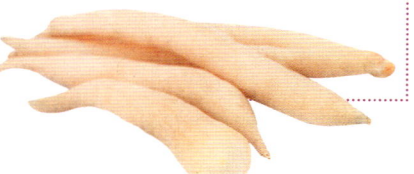

■ OATS
The B vitamins in foods such as oats, wholewheat, wholegrain rice, barley and quinoa support the adrenal glands, and can therefore help to reduce symptoms such as irritability, tension, anxiety, poor concentration and low energy,' says Henrietta Norton, nutritional therapist and founder of Wild Nutrition.

■ BROCCOLI
Cruciferous vegetables (broccoli, Brussels sprouts, watercress, cabbage and cauliflower) are especially useful for peri- and post-menopausal women. 'These vegetables contain a substance called diindolylmethane (DIM), which supports the excretion of used hormones and prevents their re-uptake,' says Fran McElwaine, health and lifestyle coach (franmac.co.uk). 'The recycling of hormones is a major factor in the hormone imbalance that creates mood swings, hot flushes and joint pains,' she says.

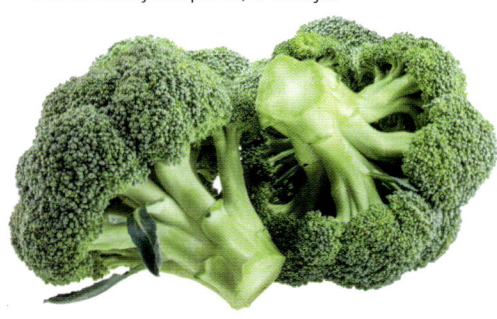

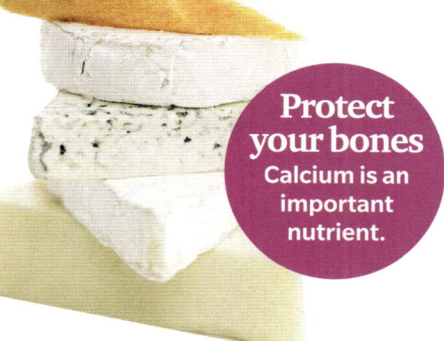

Protect your bones Calcium is an important nutrient.

■ CHEESE
Calcium is vital. 'The reduction of certain hormones causes women to start losing bone mass, which can lead to weakened bones,' says Kathy Abernethy. 'Some women may cut out calcium without realising it if they're trying to lose weight or are avoiding dairy.' Cheese, milk and yogurt are calcium-rich, as are sesame seeds, bony fish like sardines, tofu, nuts and fortified milk alternatives.

■ CHICKPEAS
'During the menopause, your oestrogen levels decrease and this can affect your muscle mass, so it's critical to make sure you're keeping up your levels of good-quality protein,' says Isabel Butler, nutritionist at Spoon Gurus. 'Legumes, like chickpeas, are a great source of plant protein to help build up muscle, and they're full of fibre to help keep your gut healthy.'

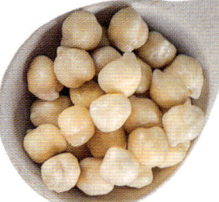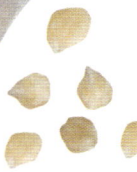

The Smart Woman's Guide to the Menopause

■ SARDINES

'Women are at a higher risk of osteoporosis due to hormone changes during the menopause, and calcium and vitamin D are two important nutrients for bone health,' explains Isabel Butler. 'Sardines contain vitamin D, calcium and omega-3, which is good for your heart and thought to help with menopause symptoms, too.'

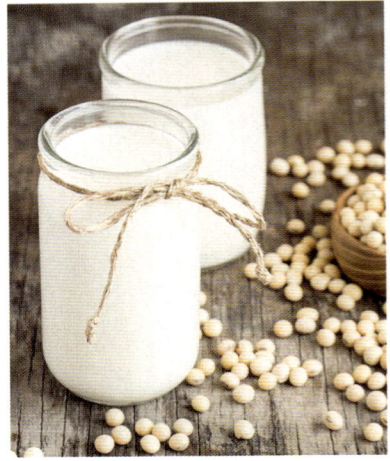

■ SOYA

Japanese women with a diet rich in soya have fewer hot flushes than Western women, according to studies, perhaps because of its high phytoestrogen content. Aim to eat two to three soya products (including soya milk, tofu, miso) per week.

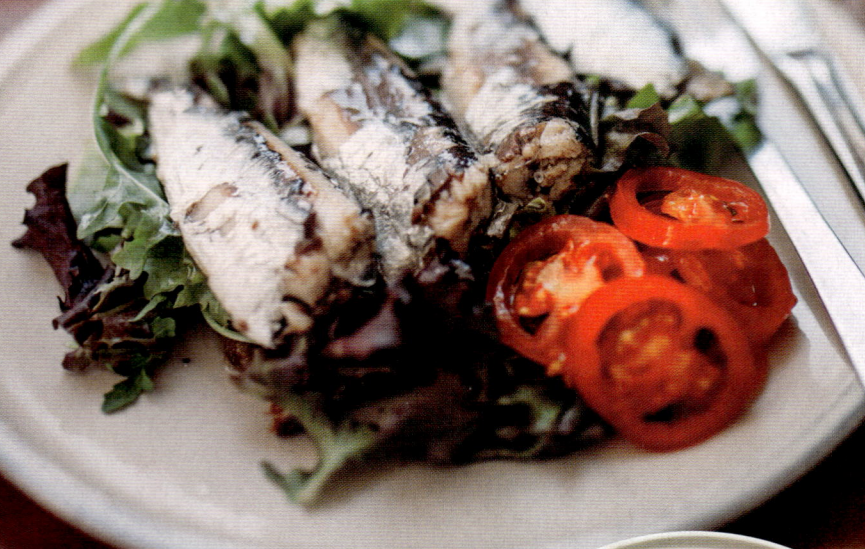

■ AVOCADO

'Healthy fats are vital for our hormonal health, as they help us make progesterone, which is one of the main female hormones supporting sex drive, sleep quality and bone health,' says women's health coach Pamela Windle. Increase your intake of healthy fats with avocados, nuts, olive oil and coconut oil.

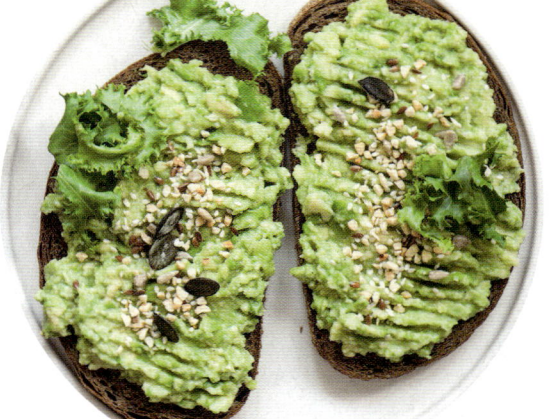

Your symptom snack chart

PALPITATIONS
'Drink water...and more water – every day,' says nutritional therapist Alison Cullen. 'It may seem boring, but it's amazingly effective. Plus cut down on caffeine, salt and refined sugar.'

NAUSEA
'Stay hydrated,' says Alison. 'Chew your food well, eat lots of cooked vegetables, and avoid white bread, pasta, rice and too many sugary foods.'

UTIs
'If you don't drink enough water, your urine will become very concentrated, irritating your bladder lining and increasing the risk of infections,' says Alison. 'Avoid coffee, tea and fizzy drinks, too.'

MOOD SWINGS
Tryptophan is an essential amino acid found in foods high in protein, such as chicken and turkey, eggs, cheese and milk. Our bodies need it to create the feel-good neurotransmitter serotonin, which promotes good mood and sleep.

INSOMNIA
The problem could be too much caffeine. Remember, it's not only in coffee and chocolate, but can also lurk in headache tablets, flavoured fizzy waters – even breakfast cereal. Check labels carefully.

TIRED ALL THE TIME
Sugar is the enemy here. 'A dramatic increase in your blood-glucose level is often followed by a crash or dip in energy, leaving you feeling tired and weak,' explains dietitian Helen Bond. 'For a sweet hit, go for fruits and nuts that give you sufficient energy to get you through the day.'

NUTRITION

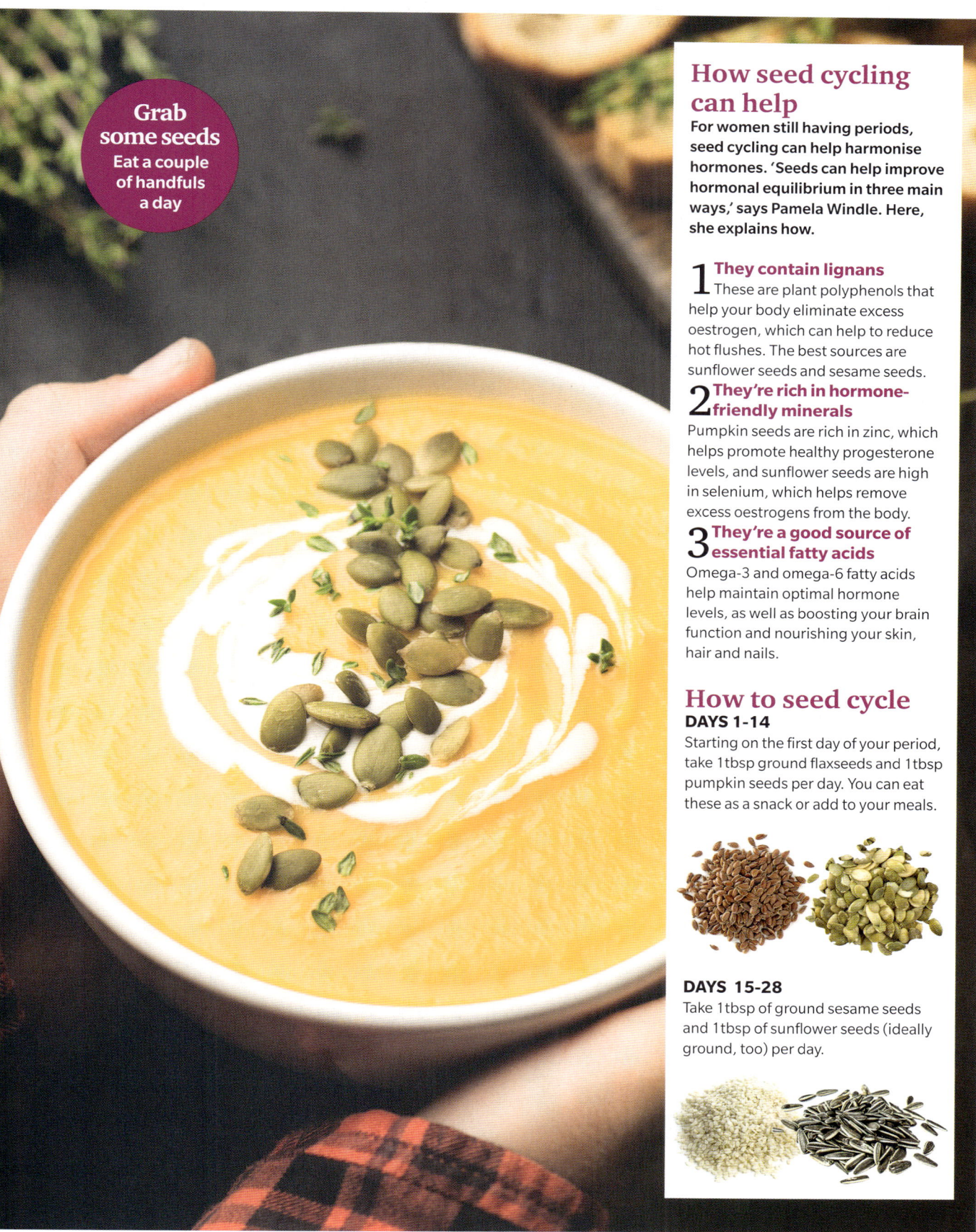

Grab some seeds
Eat a couple of handfuls a day

How seed cycling can help

For women still having periods, seed cycling can help harmonise hormones. 'Seeds can help improve hormonal equilibrium in three main ways,' says Pamela Windle. Here, she explains how.

1 They contain lignans
These are plant polyphenols that help your body eliminate excess oestrogen, which can help to reduce hot flushes. The best sources are sunflower seeds and sesame seeds.

2 They're rich in hormone-friendly minerals
Pumpkin seeds are rich in zinc, which helps promote healthy progesterone levels, and sunflower seeds are high in selenium, which helps remove excess oestrogens from the body.

3 They're a good source of essential fatty acids
Omega-3 and omega-6 fatty acids help maintain optimal hormone levels, as well as boosting your brain function and nourishing your skin, hair and nails.

How to seed cycle

DAYS 1-14
Starting on the first day of your period, take 1tbsp ground flaxseeds and 1tbsp pumpkin seeds per day. You can eat these as a snack or add to your meals.

DAYS 15-28
Take 1tbsp of ground sesame seeds and 1tbsp of sunflower seeds (ideally ground, too) per day.

The Smart Woman's Guide to the Menopause

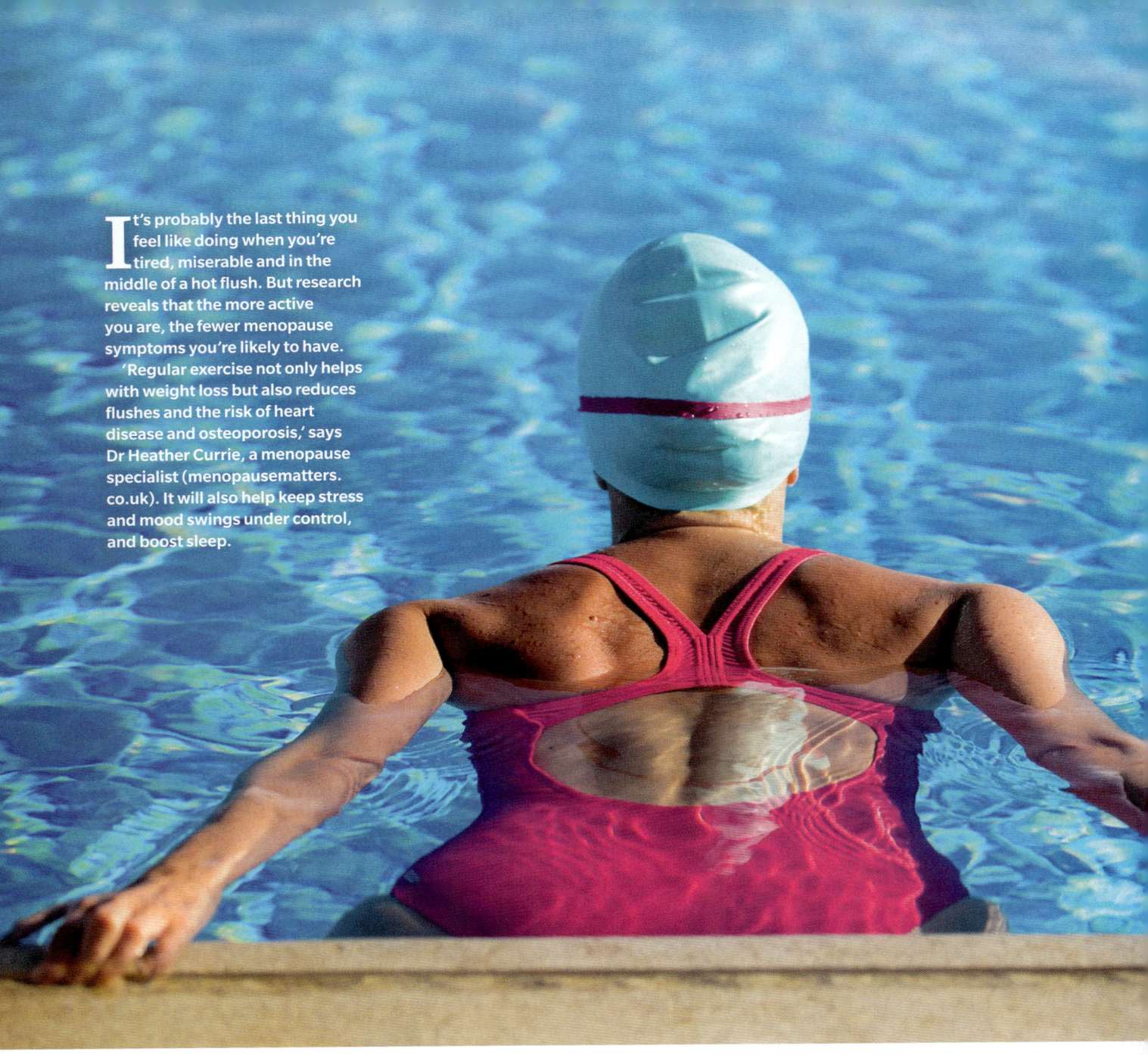

It's probably the last thing you feel like doing when you're tired, miserable and in the middle of a hot flush. But research reveals that the more active you are, the fewer menopause symptoms you're likely to have.

'Regular exercise not only helps with weight loss but also reduces flushes and the risk of heart disease and osteoporosis,' says Dr Heather Currie, a menopause specialist (menopausematters.co.uk). It will also help keep stress and mood swings under control, and boost sleep.

Ease your symptoms with exercise

Don't be beaten by the menopause. Get your body moving and show it who's boss…

EXERCISE

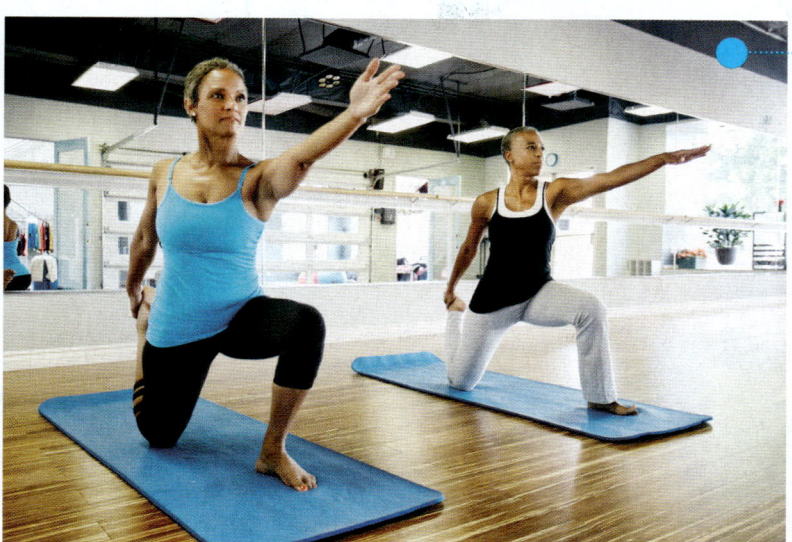

YOGA to benefit low libido
If the menopause has affected your sex drive, there's good news. 'Certain yoga poses can increase circulation to the pelvic area, which improves arousal,' says health coach Mary Nash. 'Stretches around the inner thighs can create a sense of openness, while deep tension release in and around the hips can ensure greater intimacy. There's even the Kama Sutra Eagle pose, which drives blood flow to the cervix.' For more info on how yoga can help with menopausal symptoms, contact the British Council for Yoga Therapy (bcyt.co.uk), which lists organisations whose members are yoga therapists.

SWIM to boost your mood
Research shows swimming can help with hot flushes, as the water is cooling, soothing and calming, and it boosts your mood. It's a perfect low-impact exercise, too, that can reduce the risk of heart disease, type 2 diabetes and stroke. It is also a fantastic way to keep active if you have joint or mobility problems. Start gradually (twice a week), building up the distance you swim slowly. Take a look at swimming.org/go/get-started for more information.

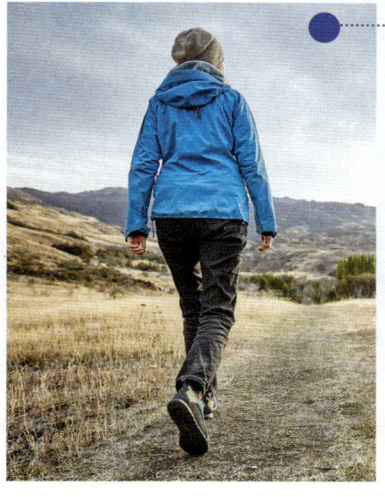

WALK for hot flushes and anxiety
'If you're feeling stressed, you're more likely to get hot flushes,' says Mary. 'Walking can help to calm the mind and body. Running can also make a difference but, for some women, it can make them feel worse. Or try HIIT (high intensity interval training) or team sports, but make sure that it's something that you really enjoy and can fit in regularly.'

Keep active
Make sure it's something you enjoy and can do regularly

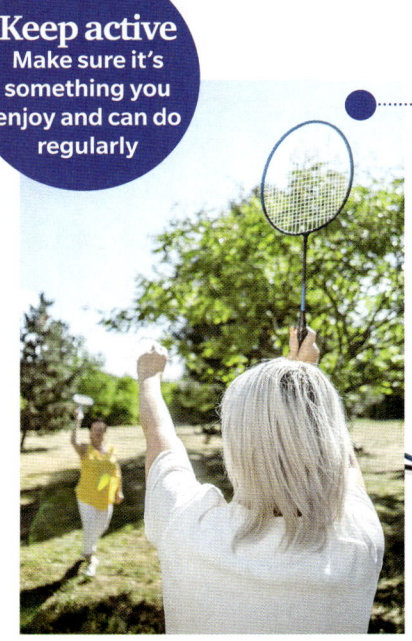

BADMINTON to banish brain fuzz
This is a brilliant way to keep your entire body strong and supple, thanks to the leaping, lunging and stretching involved. It's also great for your mind, as you have to make decisions quickly, have spatial awareness and be able to problem solve. Book a court at your local leisure centre and hire the equipment to play a game with friends or join a club.

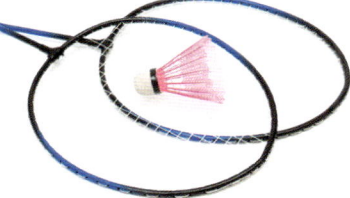

LIFT to stop muscle loss
The biggest change in your body during menopause is the loss of lean muscle and increase in body fat, especially around your waist. This is due to falling levels of oestrogen. Resistance training will help boost your metabolism, burn calories and zap tummy fat. Resistance training exercise will reduce your risk of osteoporosis, too. You can use strength bands, dumb-bells or body-weight exercises (such as press-ups or squats) at home in a 20-minute workout. Or get yourself a personal trainer for a tailor-made programme (go to nrpt.co.uk for a list of trainers).

The Smart Woman's Guide to the Menopause

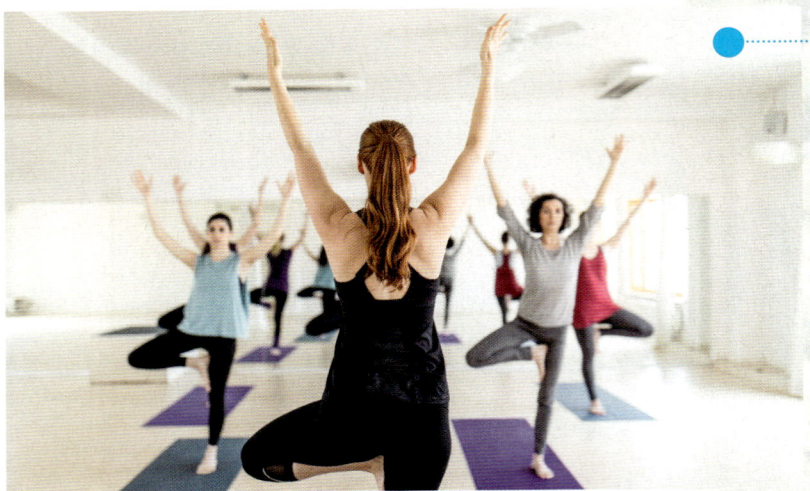

STRETCH away insomnia

Trouble sleeping? You're not alone. 'A stretching routine, such as yoga or Pilates, can reduce tension and create a sense of deep relaxation in the body, which is more conducive to slumber,' says health coach Mary Nash, who works with women struggling with menopausal symptoms. 'Alternatively, gentle stretching in the evening can help de-stress from the day and get the body ready for sleep.' Watch the beginner's guide to Pilates at nhs.uk.

Join a group It's more fun and keeps you motivated

T'AI CHI to reduce stress

Calming, meditative t'ai chi integrates body, mind and spirit. It's performed as a series of slow, graceful, controlled movements, stepping and shifting your weight, and rotating. It forces your breathing to become relaxed and deep, reducing stress and inducing a sense of calm. Find a class online near you or visit taichiunion.com.

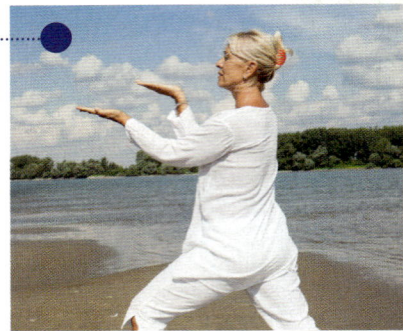

HORSE RIDE to beat the blues

Riding brings plenty of psychological, as well as physical benefits. The interaction with the horses provides a wonderful sense of wellbeing and helps relieve feelings of anxiety and stress. Being outdoors and in contact with nature also provides a feel-good factor and the all-important boost of vitamin D. Physically, horse riding is considered a 'moderate' activity so will burn calories and tone your muscles, especially in your legs and bum. Get involved in mucking out and grooming for a supercharged workout. If you're a beginner, have lessons at your local stables. In time, you'll be able to enjoy hacking in the countryside. Aim to ride three times a week for the most benefit.

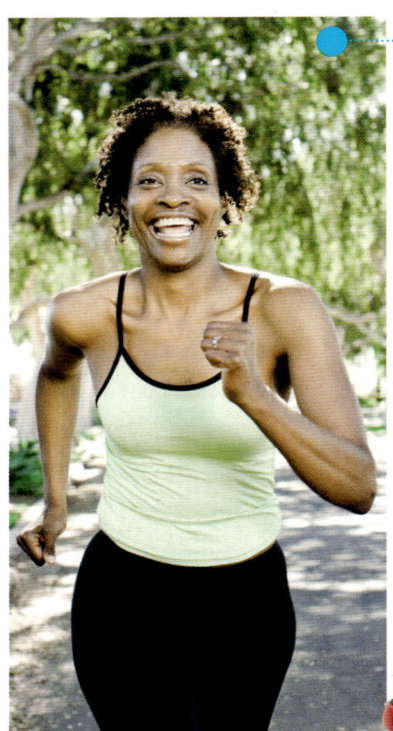

RUN off the weight

Many women take up running for the first time in their 40s and 50s. It burns more calories than any other activity and is one of the best stress busters and bone builders. Start by running twice a week for 15 minutes. Warm up by walking for two minutes, then jog at an easy 'chatting' pace for a minute, and walk for a minute. Repeat this one-minute walk, one-minute jog sequence for 15 minutes, then spend five minutes walking to cool down. Build it up by lengthening the jogs and shortening the walks and increase the total time to 30 minutes. Buy decent running shoes and a good bra. Find a group for beginners near you at parkrun.org.uk. After six months, you can increase your running sessions to three times a week.

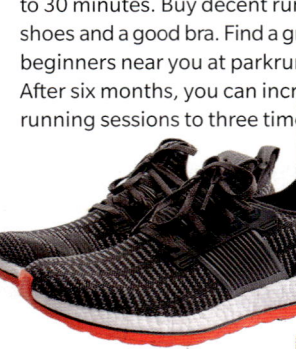

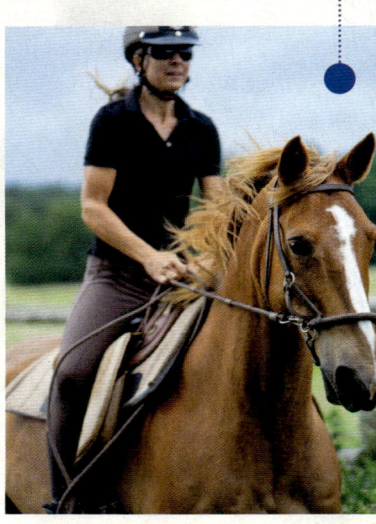

68 The Smart Woman's Guide to the Menopause

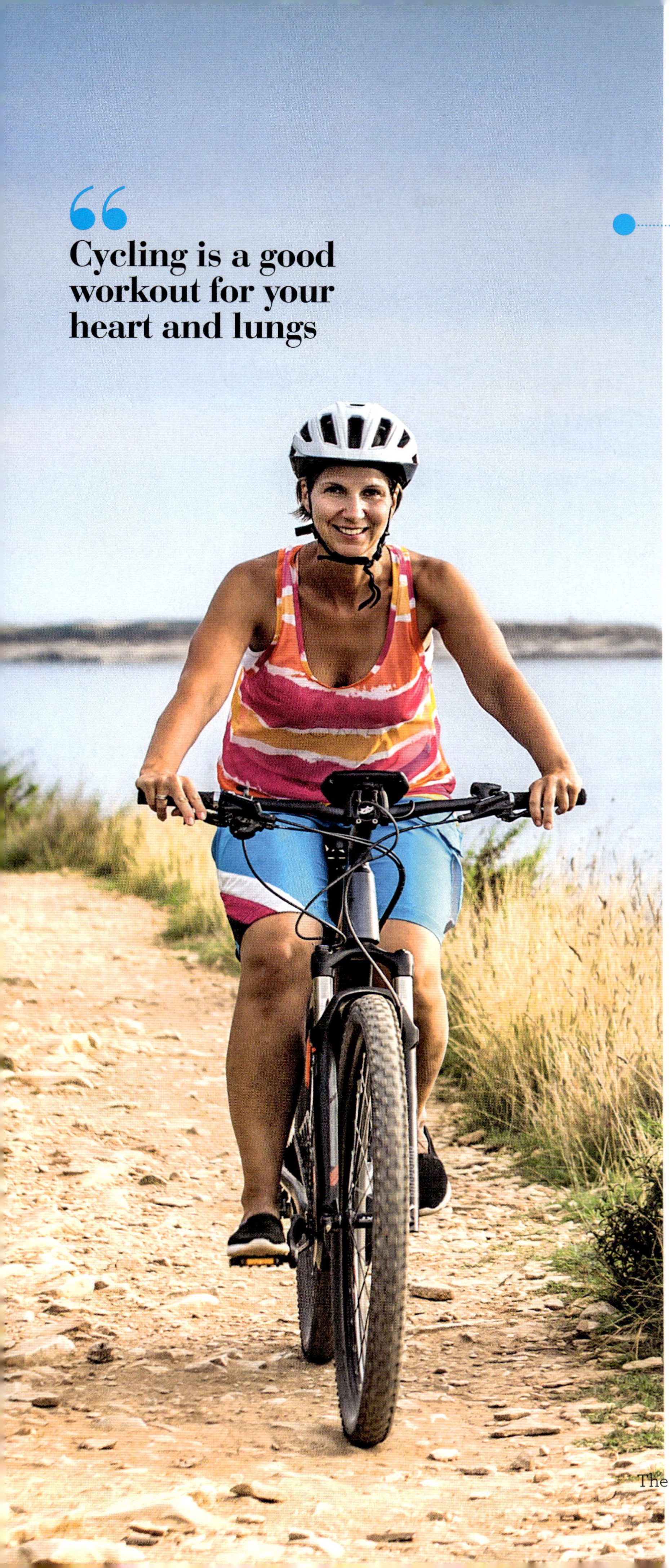

EXERCISE

> **Cycling is a good workout for your heart and lungs**

CYCLE to heart health
Cycling is a great way to build strength in your legs and tone your behind, without the risk of injury or joint problems. It'll give you your vitamin D fix and is a good workout for your heart and lungs. Riding through the countryside with the wind in your hair relieves anxiety and stress and can take you back to your childhood. Cycling is also a fantastic activity to do with family and friends. Breeze rides are organised female-only rides aimed at getting women out on bikes for the first time. Check out letsride.co.uk/breeze.

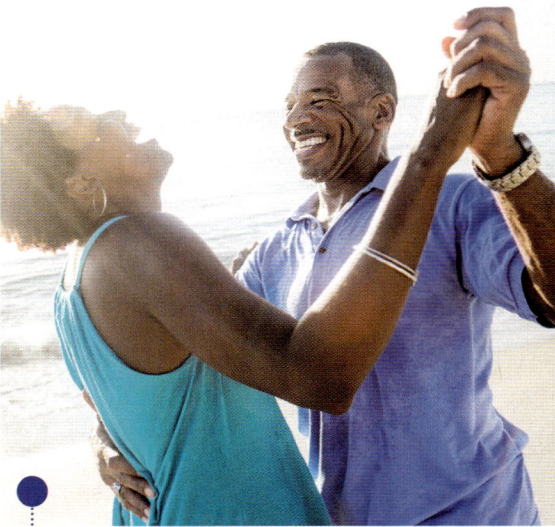

DANCE away depression
Dancing keeps you active, improves balance, posture and coordination, and as a weight-bearing activity, is great for bone health. Depending on the style and how vigorously you do it, dance can be an excellent cardiovascular workout, too. Dancing is one of the most fun and sociable ways to stay active, especially at a time when you might be struggling with low mood or depression. Try vibrant styles such as salsa, tango and ceroc, or the more exotic flamenco, pole- or belly- dancing. Check out a few different classes to see what you enjoy. Find a class or instructor at dancenearyou.co.uk which has a database of over 1,000 classes nationwide. Or look in your local paper or community magazine.

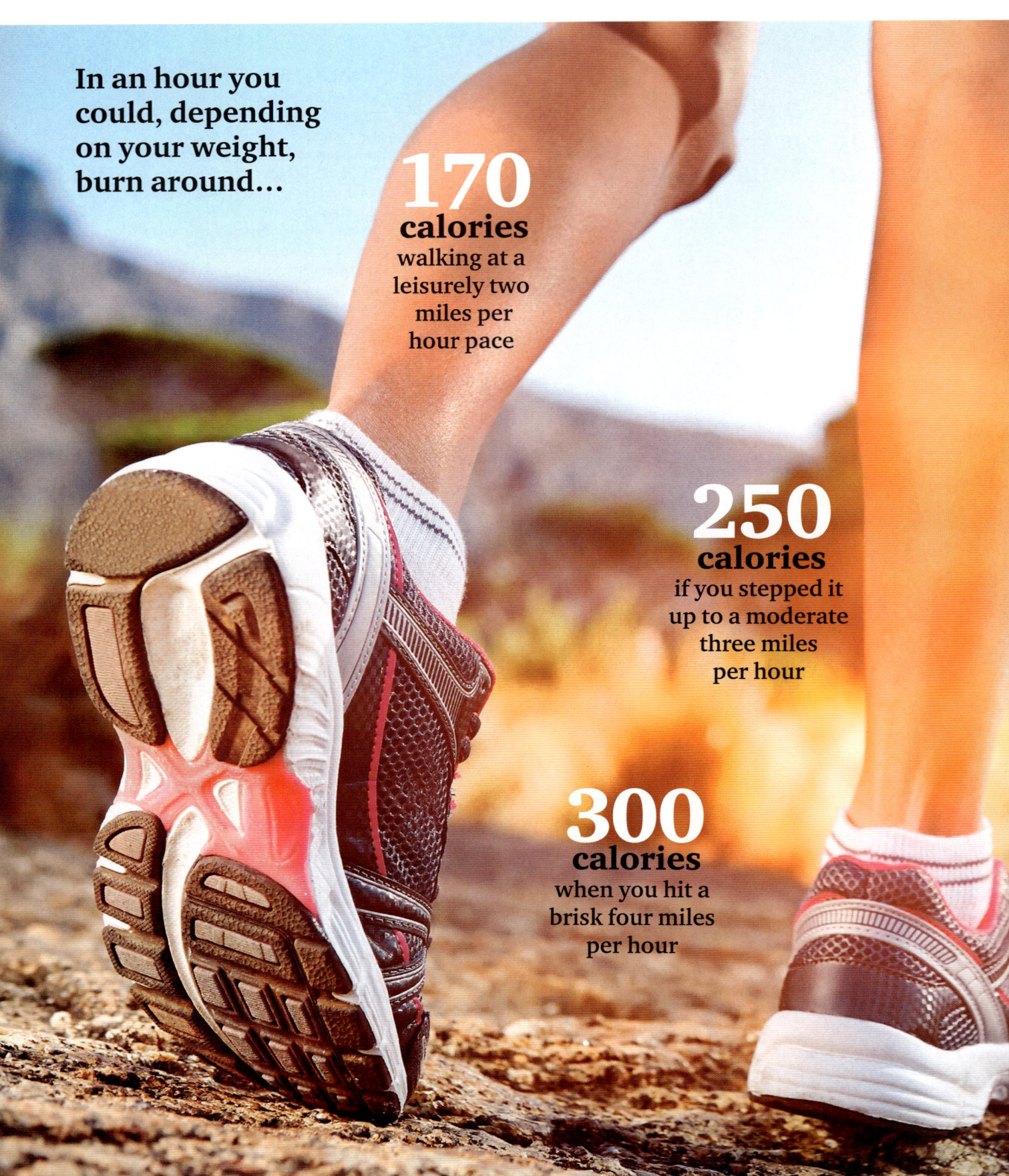

In an hour you could, depending on your weight, burn around...

170 calories walking at a leisurely two miles per hour pace

250 calories if you stepped it up to a moderate three miles per hour

300 calories when you hit a brisk four miles per hour

If you only do **one** thing...

Walk. It's free, you can do it any time, anywhere and it's the perfect answer to many menopausal miseries

How it helps your body

It's simply one of the best ways to keep you healthy – especially during the menopause. Walking lowers your blood pressure, strengthens your bones, recovers your waistline, raises your spirits and, if you start out right, it can spark a love affair with this easy way to keep fit.

➤ Reduces menopause symptoms
It particularly lessens those related to stress, anxiety and depression. Researchers found about 40 minutes' walking five times a week was when the benefit kicked in. They also found that walking can help reduce stress in postmenopausal women.

➤ Helps to regulate your hormones
Women who walk after menopause lower their risk of breast cancer – even if they do no other form of exercise – according to research by the American Cancer Society. Walking for at least an hour a day cuts risk by 14%, possibly because it regulates levels of hormones that can encourage breast tumours to grow.

➤ It's a great energy-booster
Studies have shown that if you're tired, working out at a rate of about six out of 10 for exertion is the sweet spot that makes you feel alert without leaving you feeling fatigued afterwards. A brisk walk measures about six out of 10 for effort.

➤ Feeds your brain
According to Italian research, people over 65 who used the most energy walking reduced their risk of developing dementia by 27%. It's believed that increased blood flow caused by exercise helps nourish the brain.

➤ Can cut your cravings
As well as burning 300 calories an hour, depending on your weight, a brisk 15-minute walk mid-afternoon cuts the amount of sweet stuff people consume. Researchers from the university of Exeter believe that snacking on high-calorie foods, such as chocolate, can be a mindless habit that leads to weight gain – but a short walk helped people regulate their intake by half.

Strong bones
Researchers at the US Tufts university say walkers have a slower bone-loss rate in the leg

➤ Helps fight major diseases
Walking is just as effective as running for fighting diabetes, high blood pressure and heart disease, say US researchers comparing the two groups. So long as you burn the same number of calories as a runner, you get the same benefits. That means walking for a bit longer – or a little bit faster. Try pumping your arms as you move. The faster they move, the faster your legs will go.

➤ It's a natural mood-booster
It's official – walking makes you feel better. When researchers asked people with depression to walk for 30 minutes three times a week for 16 weeks, they found it had similar mood-boosting effects to the antidepressant Zoloft.

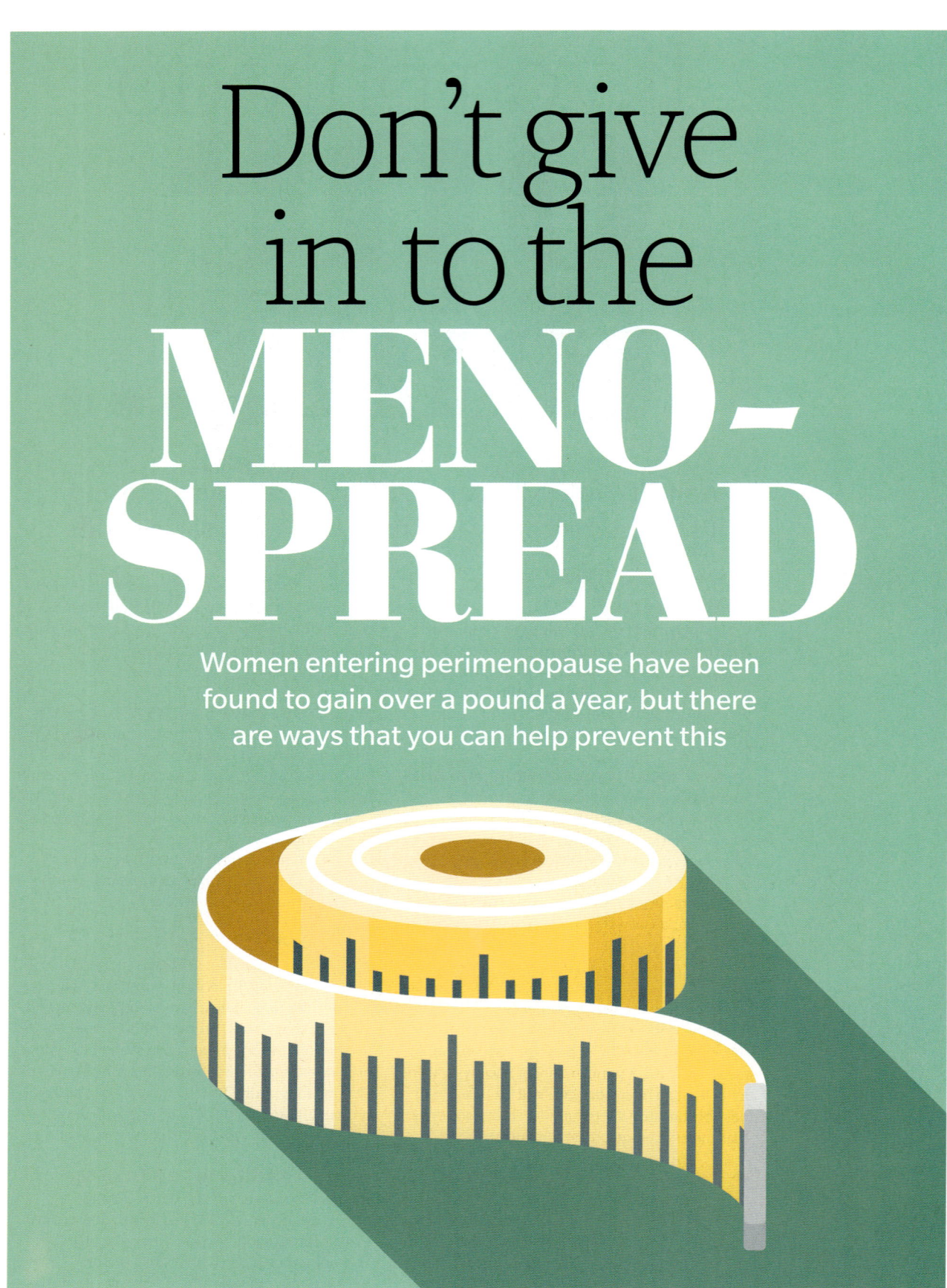

TAKE BACK CONTROL

Why do we gain weight?

Tania Adib, consultant gynaecologist at 25 Harley Street, attributes menopausal weight gain to a number of factors. 'Some of it is due to ageing. But the drop in oestrogen levels at menopause has the effect of redistributing body fat, so excess pounds tend to settle around the waist as unwelcome middle-aged spread.'
TRY *Pukka Womankind Menopause, £16.99 for 30 capsules, hollandandbarrett.com, for hormone-balancing herbal support.*

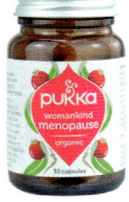

Don't overdo it
When you exercise, don't push yourself too hard, says Alison Cullen, nutritional therapist and health educator for A Vogel. 'Your body is busy, and making more demands on it will provoke a stress response that includes storing abdominal fat.'

Check your iron levels
Both haemoglobin and ferritin are important for showing iron status, especially if you've had heavy periods in perimenopause. Low iron can lead to a lack of energy, which in turn means you're less likely to exercise.

Eat mindfully
Dr Megan A. Arroll, psychologist on behalf of Healthspan, suggests that, before eating, we should ask ourselves if we're physically hungry or just craving food through boredom or stress. When eating, slow the pace by putting down cutlery between mouthfuls, and try not to eat while doing distracting activities like watching TV or working. A smaller plate can also help condition you to feel satisfied with smaller portions of food.

> **Making more demands on your body will provoke a stress response**
> *Alison Cullen*

Body and mind
Adopt a healthy diet and lifestyle to support your body through this transitional period, and try to have a positive mental attitude.

Reduce stress levels
Menopause symptoms, such as mood swings, can cause stress, which raises the level of the hormone cortisol in your body. 'When cortisol levels are high, you're more likely to develop fat around your middle,' says Alison. Get plenty of sleep and exercise, and practise meditation when possible.

Try weight training
Nicola Addison, personal trainer and Healthspan's wellbeing expert, reckons strength training is great for menopausal women. 'Insulin levels become more stable, helping with blood-sugar regulation, plus testosterone and other steroid hormones are boosted to allow for the building of more muscle.' More muscle equals less body fat. Simple.

Love kelp
Alison Cullen explains: 'Kelp is rich in minerals, especially iodine, which is important for the normal production of thyroid hormones. This, in turn, encourages your body to burn up the food you eat, giving you more energy.'
TRY *A Vogel Kelp Tablets, £7.50 for 240 tablets, avogel.co.uk.*

SWERVE...
SUGAR 'Stored as fat in the body, sugar also influences the growth of unhealthy gut bacteria, leading to increased gas formation and bloating,' says Elizabeth.
STIMULANTS Alcohol, caffeine and tobacco all lead to the release of cortisol, triggering the release and storage of glucose (sugar). Caffeine and alcohol also deplete important nutrients needed for balancing hormones and energy levels.

Fight fat with food
Include the following in your daily diet and help avoid the dreaded weight gain. A well-balanced diet, says Holland & Barrett nutritionist Elizabeth Wall, helps the body adapt to hormonal changes.

✦ **FIBRE**
Fibre binds to excess hormones to make sure they're excreted. It also helps remove toxins from the liver and colon. Ensure you eat fruit, vegetables, nuts, seeds, whole grains and legumes daily.

✦ **PHYTOESTROGEN-RICH FOODS**
They're beneficial for hormone balancing. Try eating flaxseeds, oats, soy, chickpeas and lentils. **WE LOVE:** *Holland & Barrett Natural Soya Protein Chunks, £1.99 for 375g, hollandand barrett.com.*

✦ **HERBS** Adaptogenic herbs such as Siberian ginseng and Rhodiola rosea boost immunity and help you to deal with stressful times.

✦ **BITTER FOODS** Herbal bitters (taken before meals), chicory, artichokes, rocket and radishes wake up your digestive system and help it to metabolise carbs effectively.

✦ **NUTRIENT BOOSTERS**
Vitamin C, B vitamins and magnesium help the body adapt to the stress response, as well as improving immunity and general support. Eat citrus fruits, fish, wholegrains and dark green, leafy veg.

The Smart Woman's Guide to the Menopause

Desperate to shed those extra pounds? In her book *The 21 Day Blast Plan* (HQ, £18.99), Annie Deadman – who's proudly in her midlife – has created a regime especially for women just like her. If you're looking for fat loss, new eating habits, improved health and a self-esteem boost, it's all here – and not only will you slim down, you'll sleep better, boost your energy levels and see improvements in your skin and hair. Ready for a total body overhaul? Read on…

Try this easy-to-follow healthy eating and exercise plan and see real results in just 21 days

How to ditch the menopause middle

BODY MAKEOVER

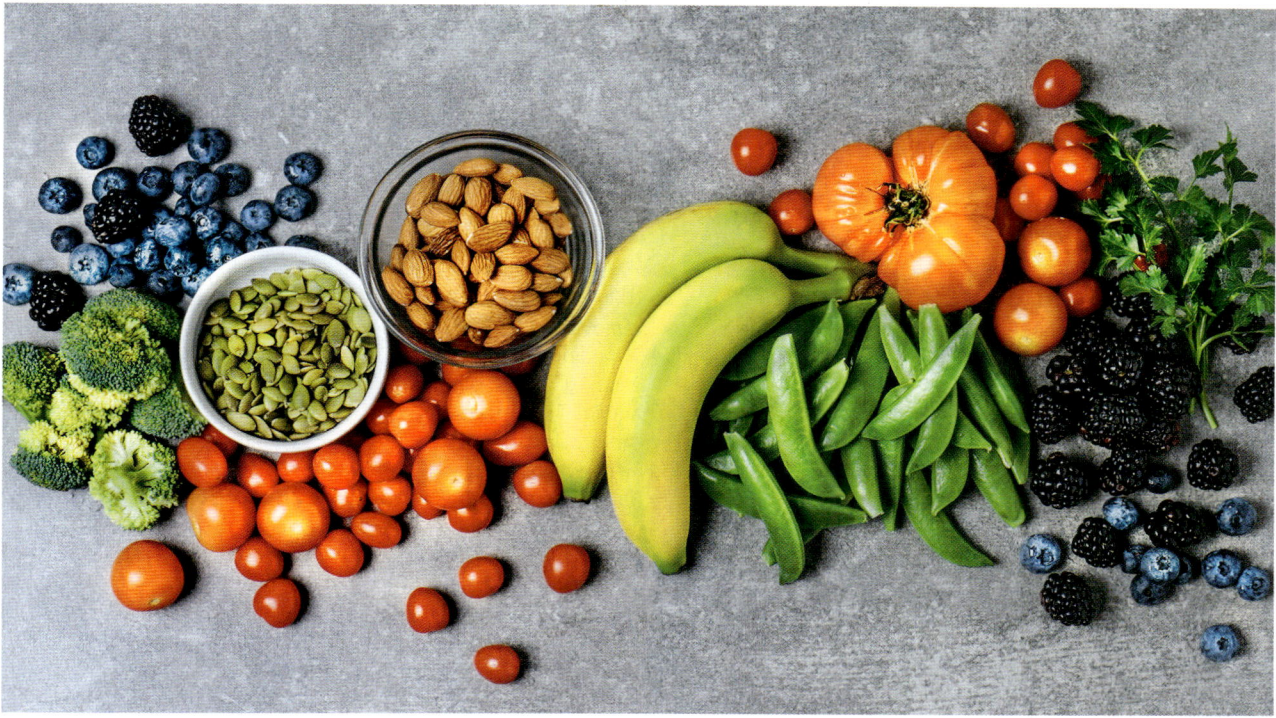

How it works

◆ **THREE MEALS** every day, plus one snack if you need it. We've included some example recipes.
◆ **PROTEIN AND FAT** Protein is important for preserving your new-found muscles, plus it keeps you full. Fats are important for taste, satiety and the goodness they bring to your body.
◆ **CARBS** You'll be eating a portion of starchy carbs, but only in the meal that follows a workout. If you work out at midday, your lunch must include carbs.
◆ **VEGETABLES** Classed as carbs, but you can pile your plate high with these.

> We want calm and balance throughout the body for this plan to work

YOUR 21-DAY FOOD LIST

The 'NO' foods
Remember, it's only for three weeks. So, in that time, try to avoid the following no-nos…
◆ **Wheat or products containing wheat.** Wheat has long been known to irritate the digestive system.
◆ **Cow's dairy.** Studies suggest it can worsen IBS, aching joints, migraines, arthritis, sinus/mucus issues, flatulence and skin disorders. There is one exception – unsweetened yogurt, which contains live cultures, good for promoting healthy gut bacteria.
◆ **Sugar.** When too much sugar is broken down into glucose in the body, it cements itself as body fat.
◆ **Caffeine.** One caffeinated drink per day is allowed. Too much caffeine increases cortisol levels, causing a hormonal imbalance. We want calm and balance throughout the body for this plan to work.
◆ **Alcohol.** It stops us losing fat, lowers our willpower and turns us into people who want to eat crisps. All. The. Time.
◆ **All processed food.** These are filled with added extras that our body doesn't agree with.

The 'YES' foods
Eat these with meals before a workout and on non-exercising days.
◆ Fresh, unprocessed meat and fish
◆ Eggs
◆ Good rusk- or gluten-free sausages
◆ Chorizo
◆ Bacon
◆ Pulses and beans
◆ Tofu
◆ Unsweetened yogurt
◆ Vegetables (apart from potatoes, sweet potatoes, butternut squash and parsnips, which are on the after-workout list)
◆ Nuts and seeds and nut butters (in moderation!)
◆ Fruit: tomatoes and avocados, plus low-carb fruits like berries, melon and peaches
◆ Protein powder (just a scoop of non-dairy)
◆ Sugar-free hot drinks
◆ Oils
◆ Water
◆ Cow's milk alternative
◆ Sauces and spices – checking first that they're sugar-free.

Only eat carbs if you've done a workout

The Smart Woman's Guide to the Menopause

The recipes

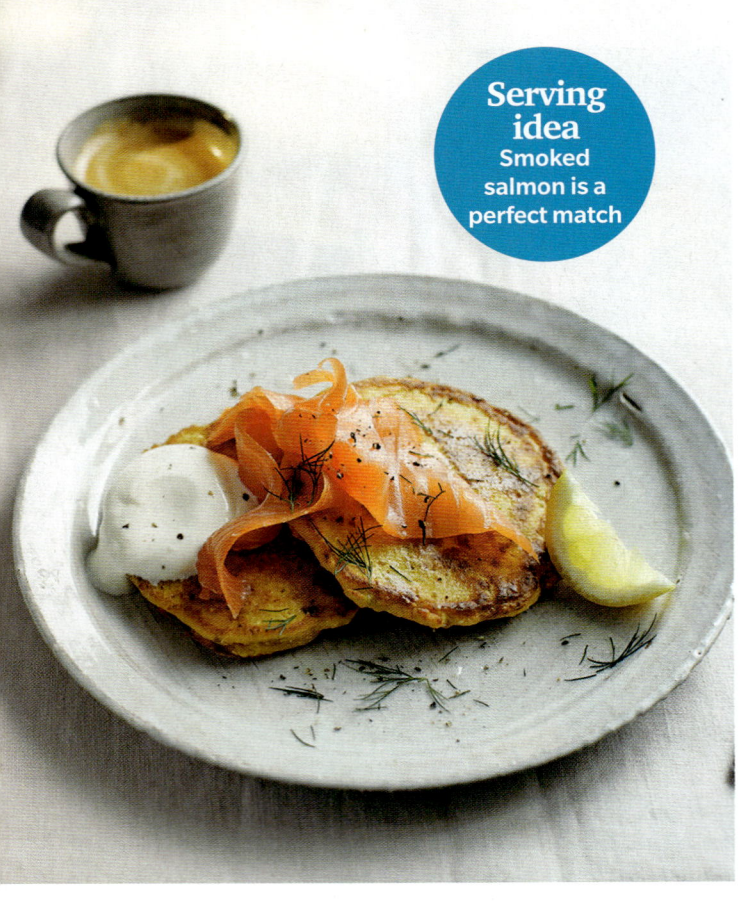

Serving idea Smoked salmon is a perfect match

BREAKFAST
Cauliflower hash browns

Serves 2 (123 cals per serving)
- 300g cauliflower, leaves removed
- 2 medium eggs
- 2 spring onions, trimmed and finely chopped
- ¼tsp ground turmeric
- ½tsp coconut or olive oil
- Salt and pepper

1 Break the cauliflower up into florets, put into a blender and process until completely broken down into a rice-like consistency.
2 Whisk eggs in a large bowl, add the cauliflower, spring onions, turmeric and seasoning.
3 Heat the oil in a large frying pan and, when hot, spoon in 4 large spoonfuls of the hash brown mixture.
4 Cook over medium heat for 4-5 minutes until golden underneath, then carefully turn over and cook for a further 3-4 minutes.
5 Serve with a protein, such as a dollop of Greek yogurt.

OTHER BREAKFAST OPTIONS
- Two rashers of grilled back bacon, a fried egg, a handful of mushrooms and two tomatoes sautéed in a teaspoon of oil.
- 200g Greek yogurt, a handful of your favourite berries and 10-15 almonds.

LUNCH
Lemon-and-olive chicken traybake

Serves 4 (311 cals per serving)
- 8 chicken thighs, skin on
- 8 shallots
- 1 red pepper, deseeded and chopped
- 1 yellow pepper, deseeded and chopped
- 50g bacon lardons
- 1 lemon, cut into wedges
- 3-4 sprigs of thyme
- 1tbsp olive oil
- 50g black olives, stoned and halved
- 300ml chicken stock
- Salt and pepper
- Steamed green veg, to serve

1 Preheat oven to 200C/Gas 6.
2 Place the chicken, shallots, peppers, bacon lardons, lemon and thyme sprigs in a large roasting tin. Drizzle with olive oil, season, then bake for 30 minutes.
3 Stir in the olives, pour over the stock and bake for a further 10-12 minutes until the chicken is cooked through and golden.
4 Serve with steamed greens or any other vegetables that need using up.

OTHER LUNCH OPTIONS
- Stir-fried vegetables with chicken, prawn or strips of beef.
- Tuna with half a can of cannellini beans, a spoonful of capers, chopped red onion, lettuce leaves tossed with some oil, lemon juice and fresh coriander.

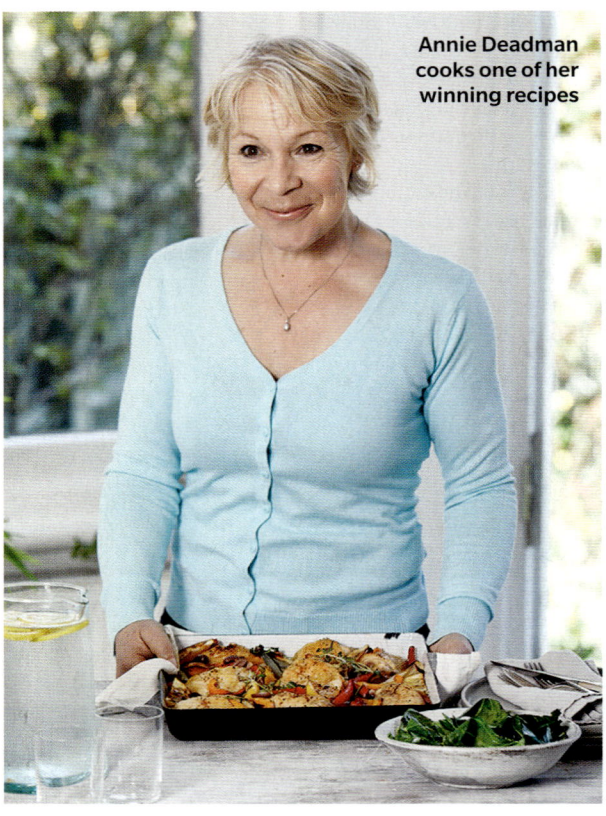

Annie Deadman cooks one of her winning recipes

76 The Smart Woman's Guide to the Menopause

BODY MAKEOVER

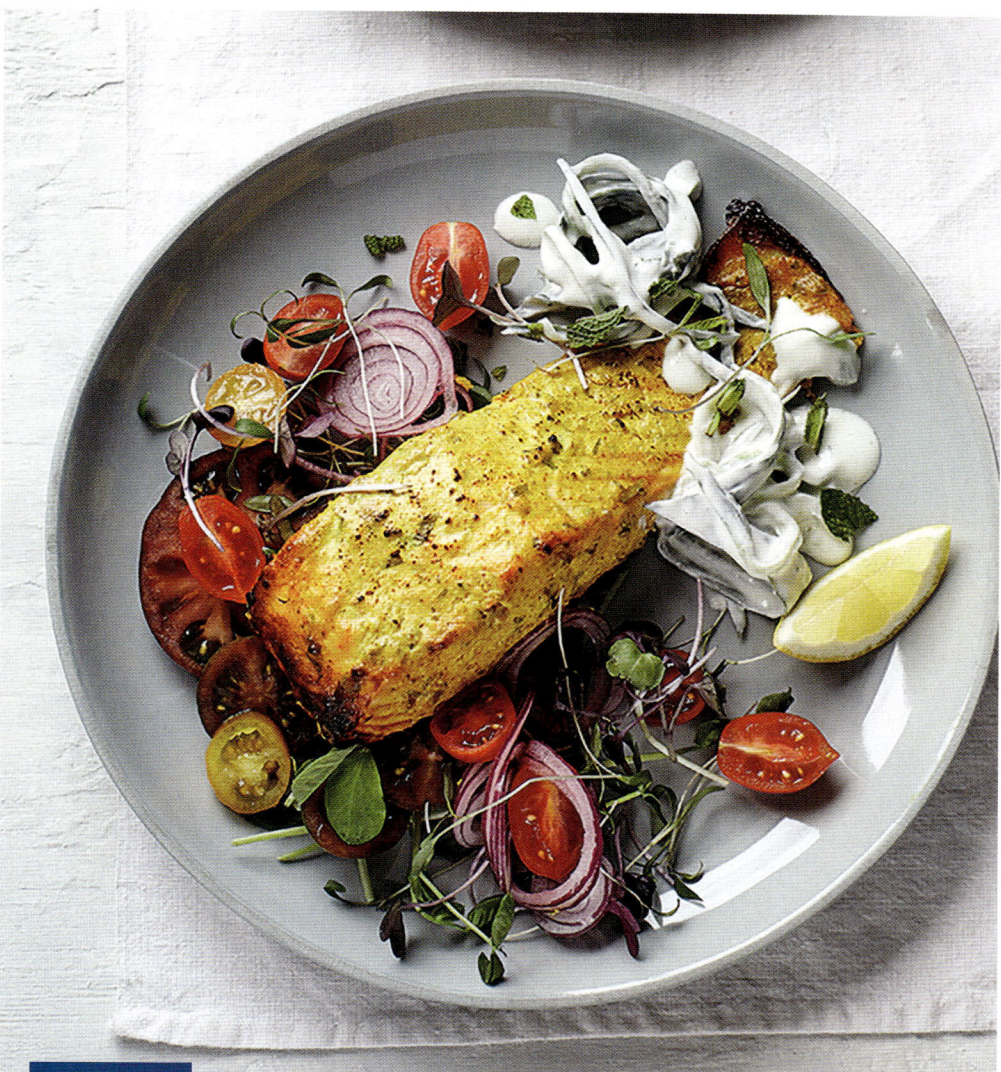

DINNER
Salmon tandoori with cucumber raita

Serves 4 (326 cals per serving)
- 200g Greek yogurt
- ½tsp smoked paprika
- ½tsp ground turmeric
- ½tsp garam masala
- ½ green chilli, deseeded and diced
- 1 garlic clove, crushed
- 1cm piece of fresh ginger, peeled and grated
- 1tbsp chopped coriander
- Juice of ½ lemon
- 4 x 150g salmon fillets
- ¼ cucumber, grated
- Small handful of mint leaves, chopped
- Vegetables or tomato and red onion salad, to serve

1. Preheat the oven to 200C/Gas 6. Pour half the Greek yogurt into a bowl. Stir in the spices, chilli, garlic, ginger, coriander and lemon juice.
2. Spread the marinade over the salmon fillets, cover and set aside for 20 minutes.
3. Mix together remaining yogurt, grated cucumber and chopped mint to make the raita.
4. Arrange the salmon fillets on a baking tray, pop into the oven and bake for 8-10 minutes until the fish is cooked through.
5. Serve with tomato and red onion salad or cooked vegetables with some bite – such as broccoli and green beans – all with a dollop of raita.

OTHER DINNER OPTIONS
- Roast dinner (but no potatoes, parsnips or Yorkshires) with carrots, peas, broccoli and greens.
- Beef (or turkey) mince, dry-fried with onion and spices, and topped with yogurt and fresh herbs, served with green veg.

After workout
- Leftover rice fried up with diced chicken, bacon, mushrooms and wilted spinach.
- Large jacket potato with a portion of beef bolognese on top.
- Bacon, egg, sausage, mushrooms, wilted spinach and some new potatoes.
- Warm quinoa, onion, garlic, herbs and chopped vegetables, sprinkled with toasted almonds.

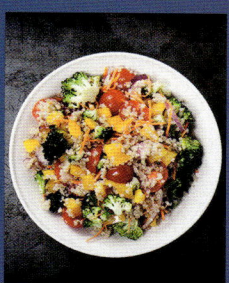

Snack right
Choose one per day, (if you need it)
- Small bowl of Greek yogurt, raspberries and coconut flakes.
- Hard-boiled eggs and cucumber sticks.
- 1tsp peanut butter mixed into Greek yogurt with celery sticks.
- Any amount of vegetable sticks.
- Slice of turkey spread with houmous and wrapped around some red pepper slices.
- Prosciutto-wrapped asparagus spears.

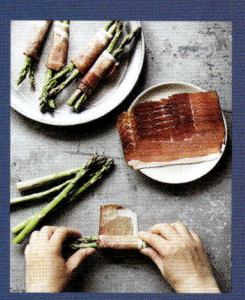

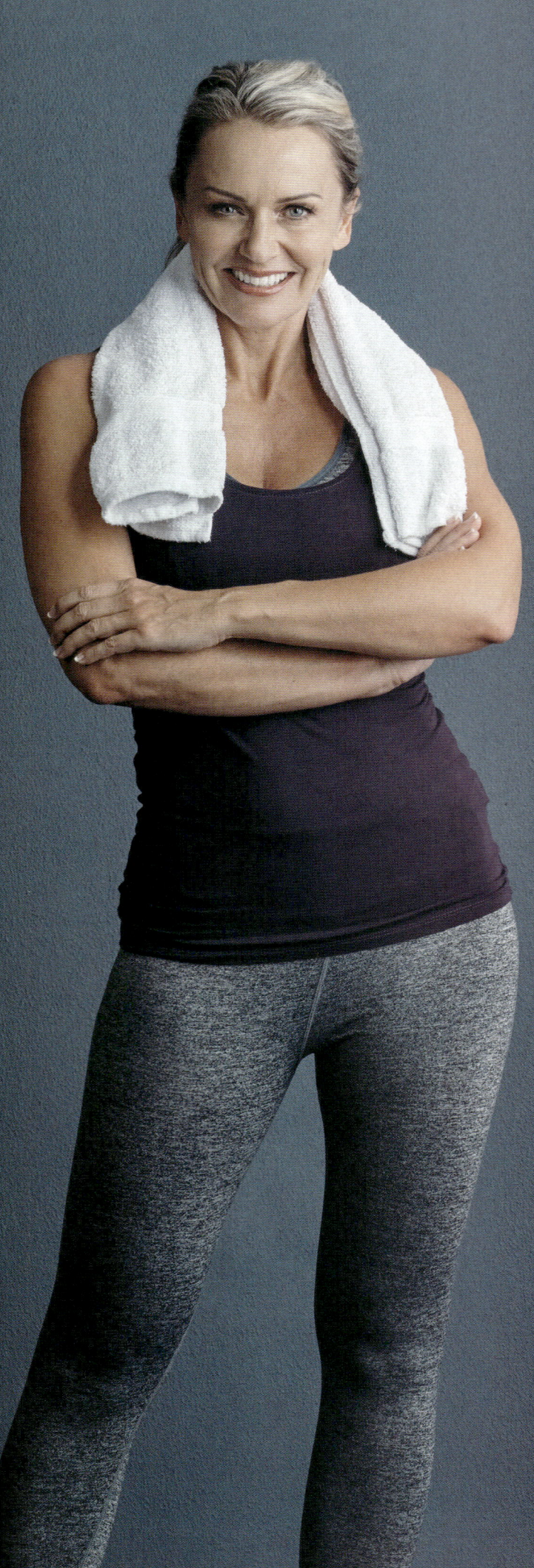

The workouts

What level are you?

NEWBIE Someone who finds climbing, say, three flights of stairs, pretty tough on the legs and lungs.
PRO Someone who is already doing some strength and fitness work, or who runs, swims or cycles regularly.

Keep to your level Don't overdo it or you'll feel defeated

Don't forget
Make sure you spend a few minutes warming up and stretching. After your workout, allow time to cool down – maybe take a slow walk around the room.

The exercise plan
✦ All you need is a timer (your phone should have one), some water and a towel.
✦ Pick your level and give this full body workout a go:

9 EXERCISES	NEWBIES 21 MINS	PRO 25 MINS
SUMO SQUATS	14 reps	20 reps
REVERSE LUNGES	14 reps	20 reps
HIGH KNEES	20 seconds	30 seconds
PRESS-UPS	14 reps	18 reps
ABDOMINAL CRUNCHES	20 reps	30 reps
SQUAT JACKS	20 seconds	30 seconds
SUPERMAN PLANK	10 reps	14 reps
DEADBUGS	10 reps	14 reps
STAR JUMPS	20 seconds	30 seconds

Rest 20 seconds between each exercise. Repeat three times.

BODY MAKEOVER

The moves

HIGH KNEES
Sprinting on the spot, but bring knees up towards chest. Pump your arms, too.

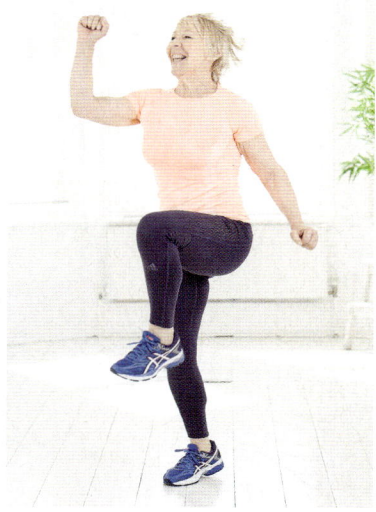

DEADBUGS
Lie on back, legs stretched out and arms above head. Keeping limbs straight, bring one leg up to meet opposite arm, as well as head and shoulders, exhaling as you do. Return to start position – flat out. Straighten up, then repeat on the other side.

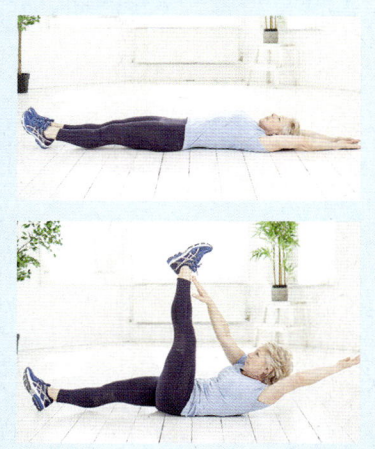

REVERSE LUNGES
Stand with feet shoulder-width apart and take a big step backwards with one leg, bending both knees. Push front foot into ground to bring back leg back to starting position. Repeat with other leg.

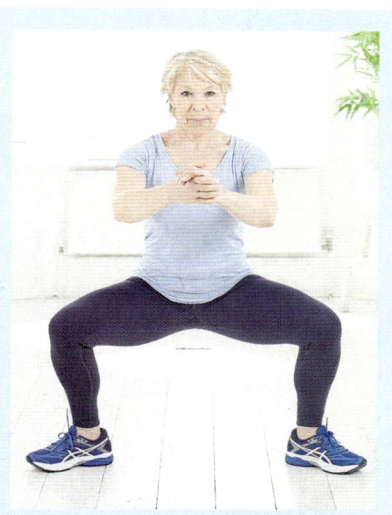

SUMO SQUATS
Stand tall, feet wider than shoulder width. Turn out feet. Keep back straight and knees facing same direction as toes, lower yourself to the floor, then squeeze glutes (bottom) to bring you back up.

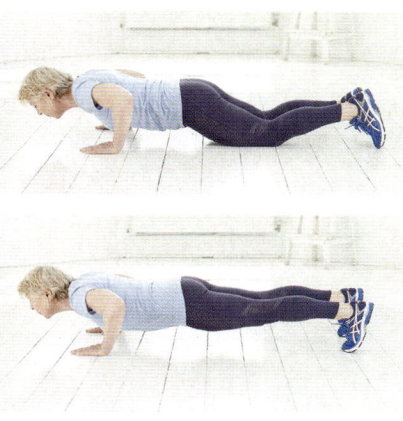

PRESS-UPS
Start on all fours, hands slightly wider than shoulder-width. Lower upper body to floor, keeping head beyond hands, not in between. To come back up, exhale and push floor away from you. Make it harder by doing this with knees off the floor.

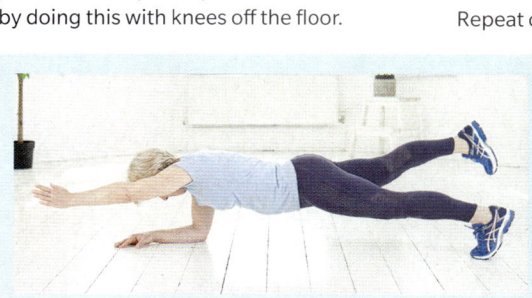

ABDOMINAL CRUNCHES
Lie on back, knees bent, feet flat on floor. Bring hands behind head, overlapped, and bring elbows forwards a little. As you breathe out, lift head and shoulders from floor and hold for a split second. Breathe in as you lower back down, then go straight back up for next rep.

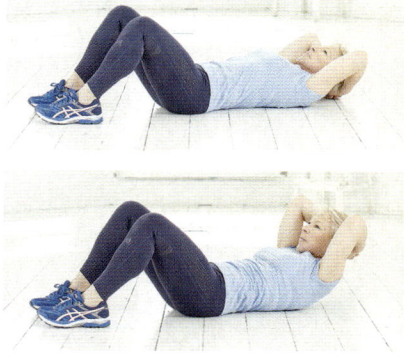

SQUAT JACKS
Stand tall, legs apart and slightly bent. Jump both legs out to side and then back, in and out but keep them slightly bent all the time.

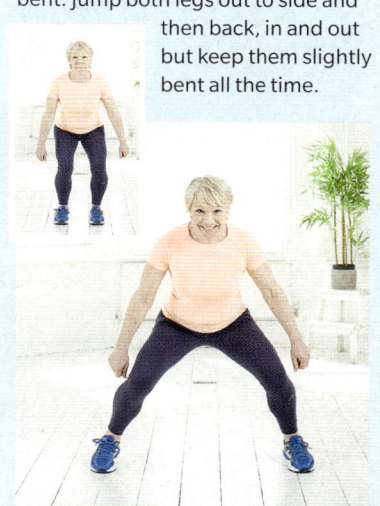

STAR JUMPS
Jump both legs out to the sides and do the same with the arms. Jump back. Repeat continuously.

SUPERMAN PLANK
On all fours, take right leg straight out behind you and extend left arm in front, level with your ear. Hold for a couple of seconds, then repeat on opposite side. Try not to move your spine or pelvis too much.

The Smart Woman's Guide to the Menopause

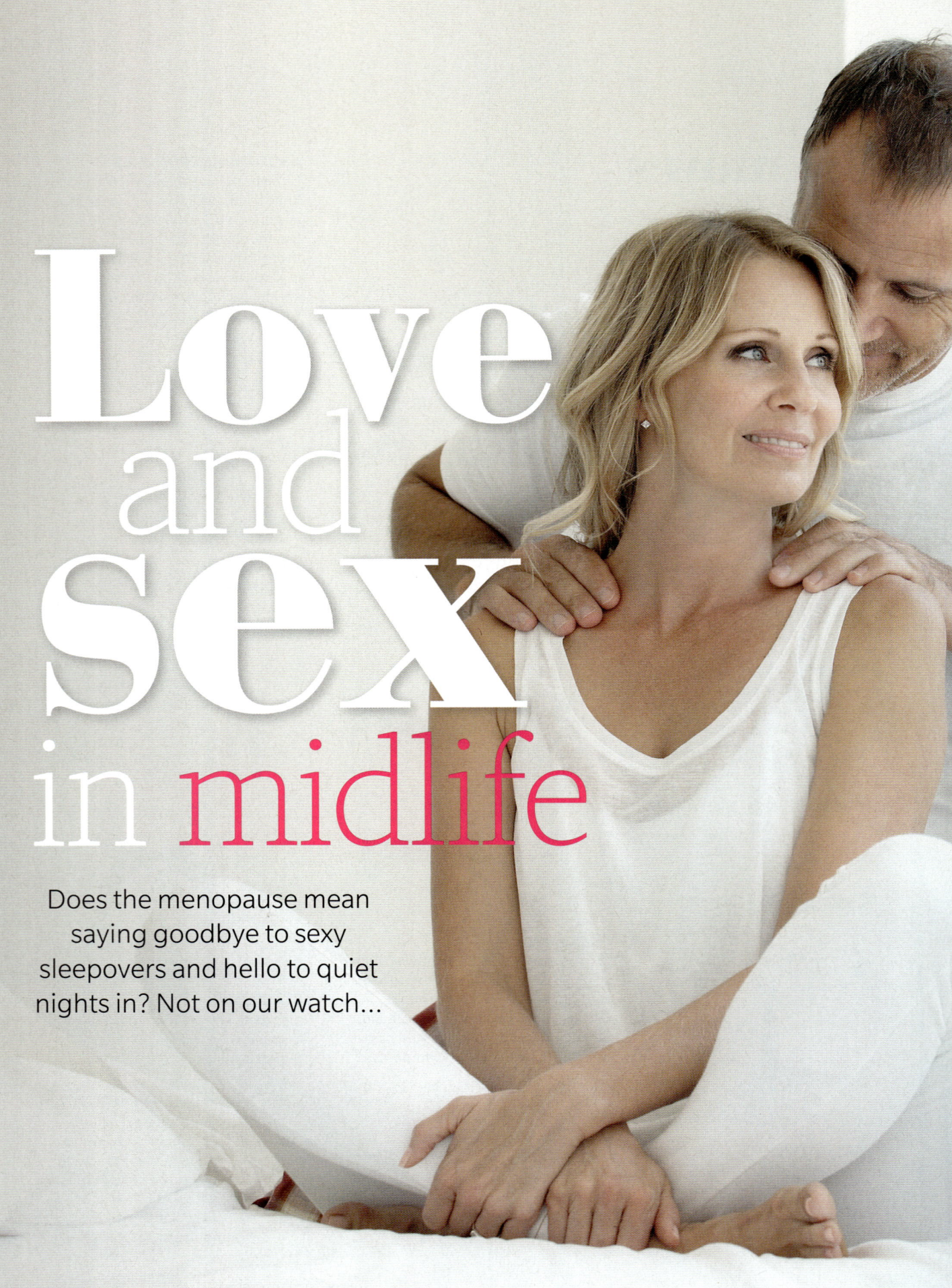

Love and sex in midlife

Does the menopause mean saying goodbye to sexy sleepovers and hello to quiet nights in? Not on our watch…

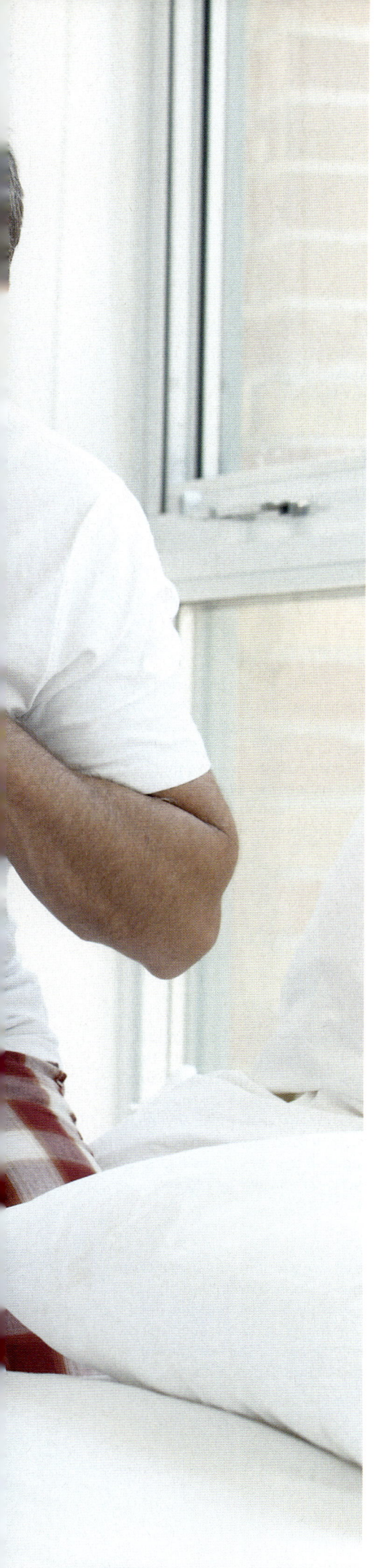

YOUR LOVE LIFE

Hitting your 50s – and the menopause – shouldn't mean a sad farewell to your sex life. 'We're living longer and staying younger at heart – 60 is definitely the new 40,' says GP Dr Sarah Brewer. 'Ever since the launch of Viagra, sex in later life has become more openly discussed, and those with falling libidos are more likely to seek help.'

Doctors are becoming more sex savvy, too. 'They're getting better at asking about the sexual side effects of medications and addressing sex after someone's been diagnosed with cancer or a stroke,' she adds.

There are many body-boosting benefits of turning up the heat with your other half, including increasing immunity, lowering stress and blood pressure and improving heart health. It can also help turn back the clock – sex stimulates the release of oestrogen and testosterone, boosting collagen and preventing hair loss.

Physical crossroads

It's not always smooth sailing, though. The menopause can have a big impact on your sex life. Levels of oestrogen and testosterone can drop significantly – the former affecting blood flow to your vagina. As a result, you may experience dryness, which can make penetration uncomfortable and reaching orgasm difficult. Bath oils and shower gels can aggravate this condition, so experts recommend washing using lukewarm water, alone or with a soap-free cleanser.

'You could try Healthspan Omega 7 Sea Buckthorn Oil supplements (£16.95 for 60 tablets),' says Dr Brewer. 'The beneficial omega-7 oils are important building blocks for healthy skin and mucous membranes.'

Don't forget lubrication – it can help maintain intimacy levels, make sex more comfortable and, in turn, boost your confidence. If a leaky bladder is making you self-conscious, Dr Brewer advises doing pelvic floor exercises, which will also boost your lovemaking experience.

Self-help
Many issues, including low self-esteem, loss of libido and lack of energy, can be helped by taking regular exercise and spending more close time with your partner.

Mental milestones

Low self-esteem can also have a knock-on effect on your sex life. Just remember – you may not still have the bottom of a 20-year-old, but it's important to celebrate your body and what you can do with it.

Low libido, which is common after the menopause, can be caused by falling oestrogen levels, tiredness, loss of confidence and stress. Regular exercise can help boost stamina, strength and self-esteem, while spending time with your partner can increase intimacy.

Stress can also have a negative impact on your sex drive, so it's worth finding a coping mechanism. 'It's important, too, that you don't feel pressured into having sex if it's not what you want,' explains Dr Brewer. 'If this causes difficulties in your relationship, you should seek professional counselling.'

✦ *Overcoming Low Sex Drive* by **Dr Sarah Brewer (£6.99, Medilance).**

The Smart Woman's Guide to the Menopause

LET'S GET IT (BACK) ON

If health problems – or simply a lack of sizzle – are holding you back in the bedroom, try these ideas to help spice things up again…

Menopause isn't a deal-breaker

Feeling drier than a cream cracker? Try **Regelle Long Lasting Vaginal Moisturiser (£16.99 for a 12-pack, regelle.co.uk).**

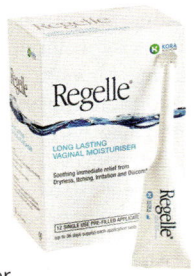

You need to put in the prep when it comes to your pelvic floor, too. 'People who can activate their pelvic floor will experience more intense orgasms,' says Dr Ruth Maher.

Add the right heat

Hot flushes left you feeling unsexy? Going back to basics can be just as good a way to connect with your partner. 'Sit on the bed facing each other and hold hands,' says romance and relationship expert Vena Ramphal (venaramphal.com). 'Look into each other's eyes for several minutes,' she advises. 'Eye gazing is very powerful.'

Start slowly

Begin with sexy texting. 'Put technology to good use,' says Vena. 'It's a fun, cheeky tease, especially if you send that text in the middle of a working day.' Just a smiley selfie or a cheeky wink emoji can help get the ball rolling. (You definitely don't have to send nude or semi-naked photos!)

Never forget foreplay

It's still possible to feel flushed with desire, however many years you've been doing it for. But how best to go about it? 'Make foreplay the main course,' says Vena, 'with lots of stroking, holding and kissing. This builds a deeper sexual and emotional connection.'

Try not to nag

So they can't stack the dishwasher or close the lid on the toothpaste – but bite your tongue, especially when you're in the bedroom, as nagging is a really big turn-off. 'Nagging subconsciously reminds your partner of being told what to do by their mother – which is one of the fastest ways to turn someone off,' says love coach Persia Lawson (persialawson.com). Leave the thought of daily life and chores at the bedroom door and save those disagreements for another time.

Tell them what you want

If you don't hold back on voicing your opinion when it comes to sorting the recycling bins, what film to watch or where to go for dinner, then don't hold back in the bedroom either. If the only way you ever reach full orgasm is through masturbation, then show them how it's done.

Zip it

Take resentment about an unresolved matter into the bedroom and you'll find it hard to switch your mindset to sex. Settle matters as and when they come up or save your discussion for later…

Embrace fantasies

They can help unlock your sex play potential. 'Fantasies are natural, healthy and have no connection to cheating,' says psychologist Emma Kenny. 'The majority of women fantasise about sex with their partner's friends, work colleagues or pretty much anyone. You don't have to tell them you're imagining their best friend on top of you – we all have our secrets.'

Change it up

We all love a routine. But if yours is same-position sex with the lights off every other Tuesday, then you need to mix things up. 'Break out of your comfort zone and start experimenting,' urges Dr Ruth Maher. Changing

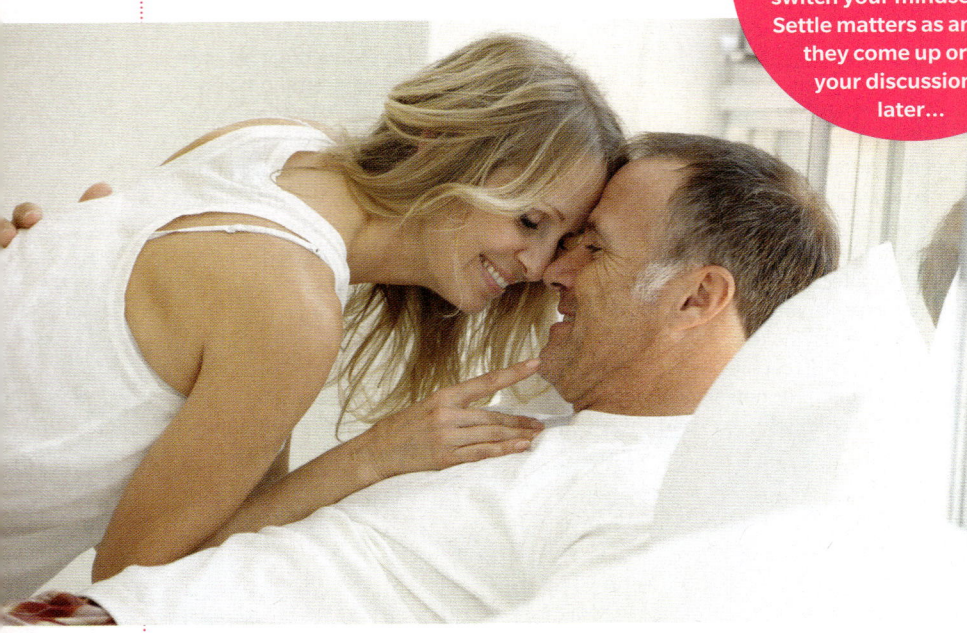

YOUR LOVE LIFE

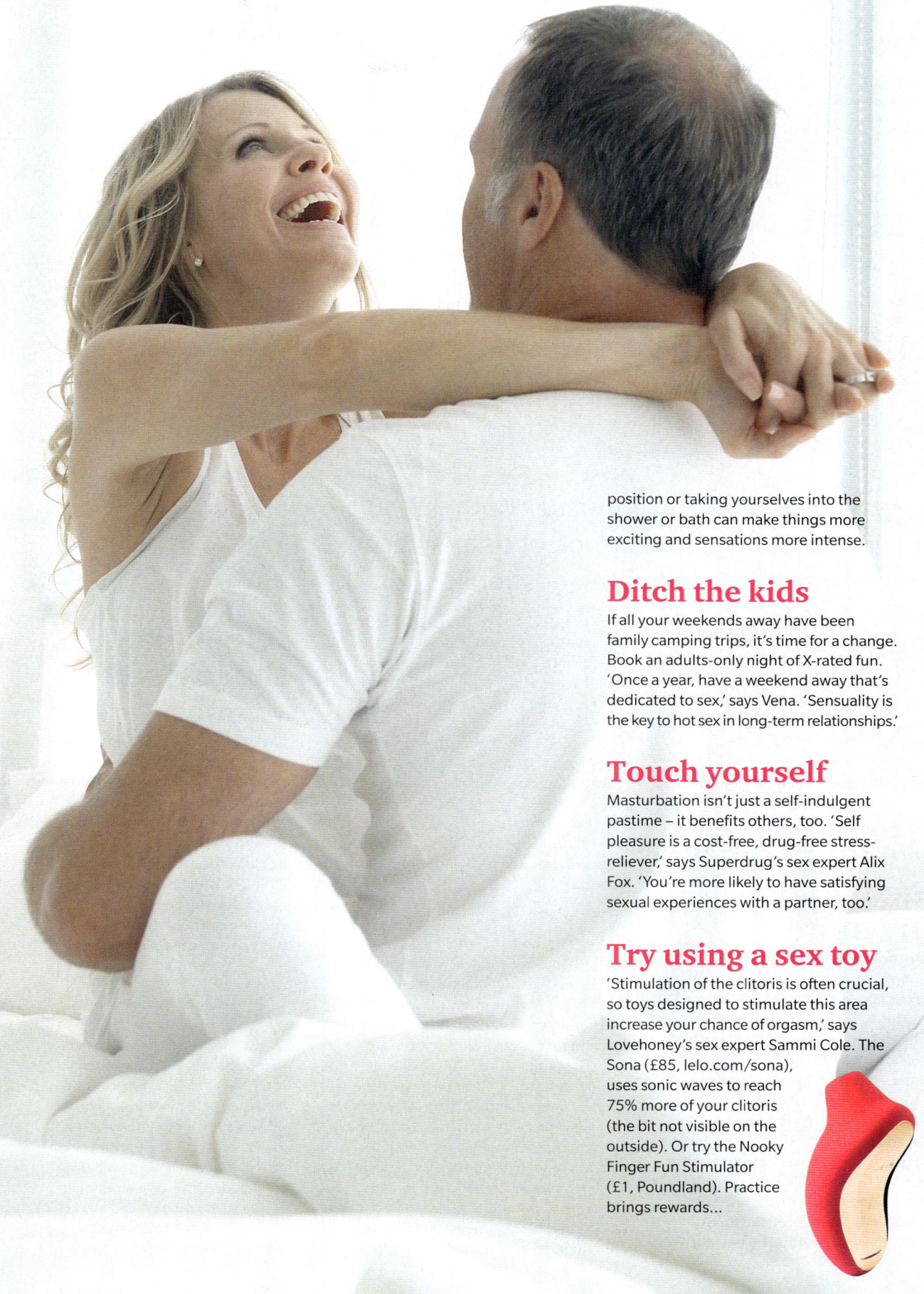

position or taking yourselves into the shower or bath can make things more exciting and sensations more intense.

Ditch the kids
If all your weekends away have been family camping trips, it's time for a change. Book an adults-only night of X-rated fun. 'Once a year, have a weekend away that's dedicated to sex,' says Vena. 'Sensuality is the key to hot sex in long-term relationships.'

Touch yourself
Masturbation isn't just a self-indulgent pastime – it benefits others, too. 'Self pleasure is a cost-free, drug-free stress-reliever,' says Superdrug's sex expert Alix Fox. 'You're more likely to have satisfying sexual experiences with a partner, too.'

Try using a sex toy
'Stimulation of the clitoris is often crucial, so toys designed to stimulate this area increase your chance of orgasm,' says Lovehoney's sex expert Sammi Cole. The Sona (£85, lelo.com/sona), uses sonic waves to reach 75% more of your clitoris (the bit not visible on the outside). Or try the Nooky Finger Fun Stimulator (£1, Poundland). Practice brings rewards…

Talking sex

Many of us find talking about sex both difficult and embarrassing, so why not let us answer some of your most intimate questions?

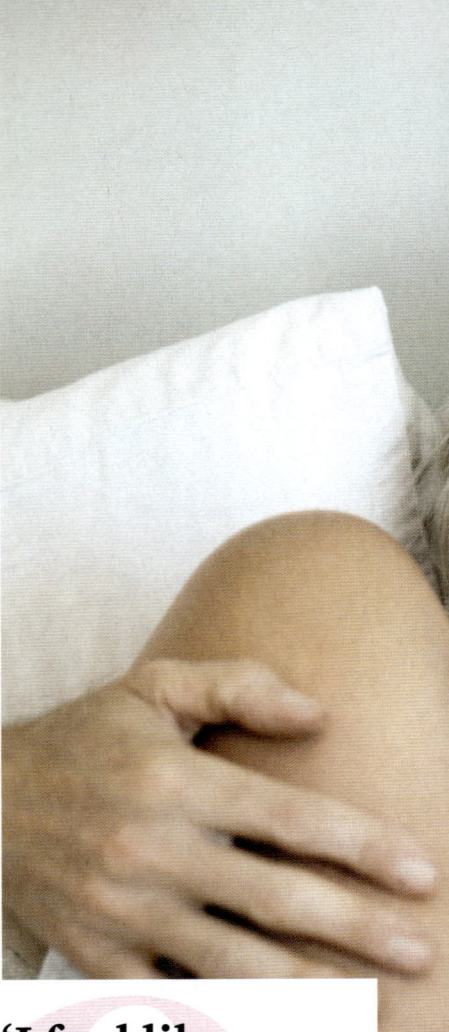

Talking to our nearest and dearest or even to close women friends about our sexual feelings, desires and behaviours is still very difficult for many of us.

Communication is important for any healthy relationship, as it allows us to share feelings and tackle problems together. This is particularly true of your sex life, especially if something is worrying you. So we hope the selection of dilemmas we've chosen to highlight will answer some of your concerns and encourage you to talk more openly with your partner about intimate issues.

'We don't fancy each other any more'

We're both in our late 50s and, since the menopause (or maybe even before), I haven't been interested in having sex. This isn't in itself a problem in our relationship because my husband feels the same way. We still love each other deeply – we seem to have a stronger relationship than many of our friends – and we cuddle up on the sofa all the time and hold each other in bed, but we just don't fancy each other any more in that way. I guess you might describe it as more of a brother-sister relationship.

I read in the papers all the time about how we should all be having rewarding sex, which makes me feel we're freaks who should be doing something about it.

A The modern world does sometimes appear to be obsessed with sex. But don't let that make you feel that you are in any way a 'freak' for choosing not to continue making love. Most research would suggest there are millions of couples in the UK who, while still in a loving relationship like you, have stopped having sex, and there is absolutely nothing wrong with that if that's what you both choose. Some of the greatest love affairs in history have been sexless, and if you've achieved a relationship where you are in tune, mutually supportive and wonderfully happy together, then you are extremely fortunate.

'I feel like the invisible woman'

I'm 54, through the menopause, and feel like the invisible woman. I'm not the woman I was – I look in the mirror and I can't bear it. My husband is the same age as me and still looks great. He says he still finds me attractive, but I think he's just being kind. He's asked me why I've stopped wearing sexy nightwear. The truth is it's because I feel so unsexy.

A You may not be the woman you were, but it doesn't mean you're not as gorgeous – if not more so. Compare yourself to a 21-year-old and you'll always feel bad. Focus on what you've got – lovely eyes, for example – listen to your husband, believe him, and start showing off your beautiful older body. Otherwise, in another 30 years, you'll look back to today and think, 'What a fool I was for thinking I wasn't still attractive!'

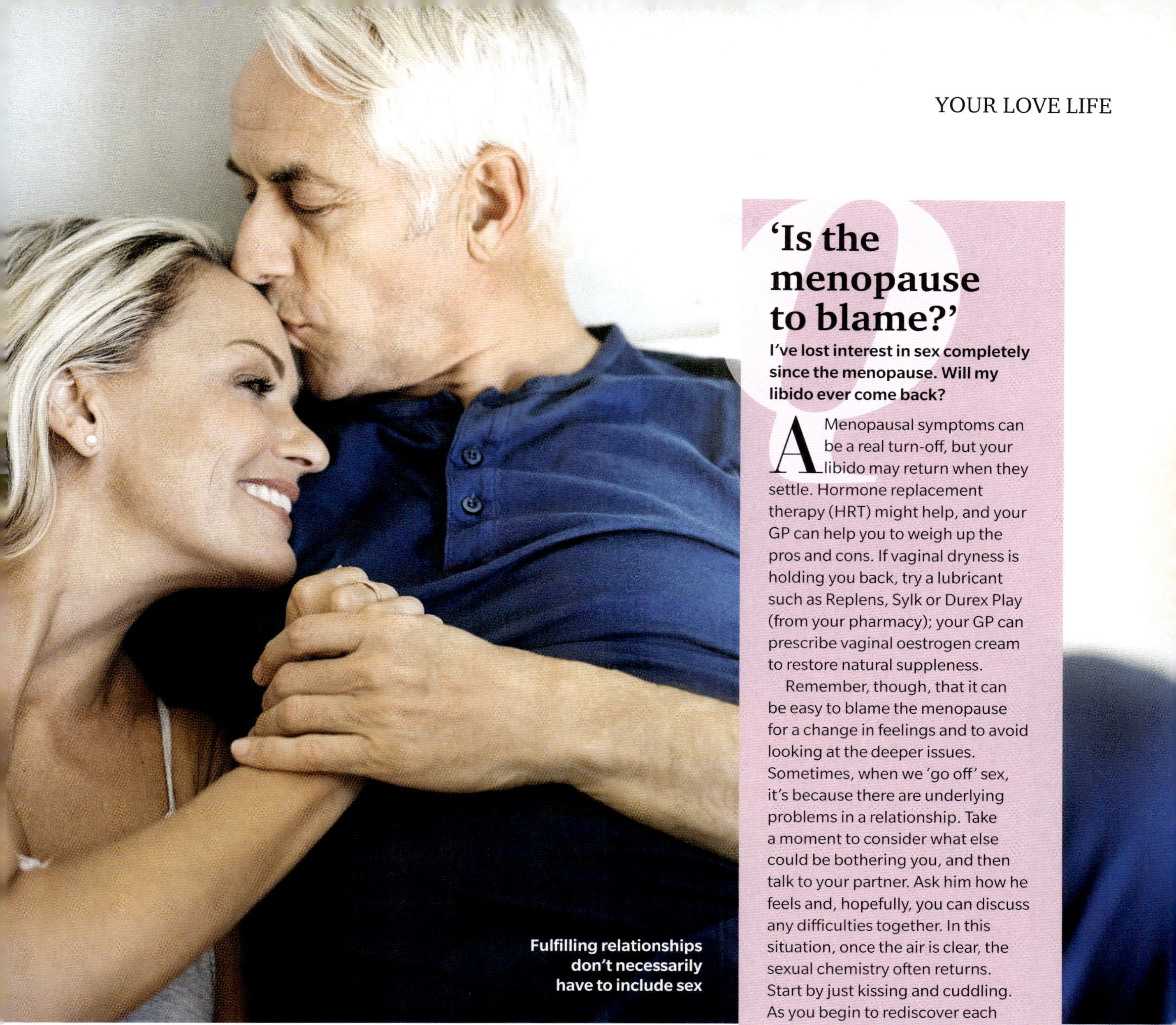

YOUR LOVE LIFE

Fulfilling relationships don't necessarily have to include sex

'Is the menopause to blame?'

I've lost interest in sex completely since the menopause. Will my libido ever come back?

A Menopausal symptoms can be a real turn-off, but your libido may return when they settle. Hormone replacement therapy (HRT) might help, and your GP can help you to weigh up the pros and cons. If vaginal dryness is holding you back, try a lubricant such as Replens, Sylk or Durex Play (from your pharmacy); your GP can prescribe vaginal oestrogen cream to restore natural suppleness.

Remember, though, that it can be easy to blame the menopause for a change in feelings and to avoid looking at the deeper issues. Sometimes, when we 'go off' sex, it's because there are underlying problems in a relationship. Take a moment to consider what else could be bothering you, and then talk to your partner. Ask him how he feels and, hopefully, you can discuss any difficulties together. In this situation, once the air is clear, the sexual chemistry often returns. Start by just kissing and cuddling. As you begin to rediscover each other, you're likely to find yourself becoming sexually aroused.

However, it does happen that some couples are happy to say goodbye to a sex life after a certain point in life. There's no law which says we have to go on having sex to the very end of our days – and, if that's the way you feel, then, of course, that's also fine.

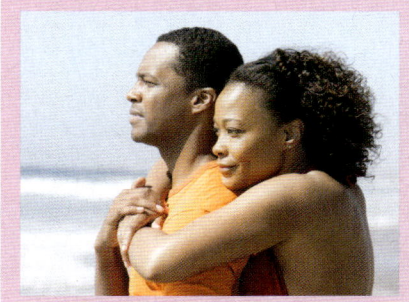

'Is it OK to be more adventurous?'

My friend took me to an Ann Summers party. I've never seen such things! I knew about vibrators (not that I could imagine using one) but not about nipple clamps or couple massagers. Some of them really turned me on, so is there anything wrong with wanting to try them?

A Of course not, as long as both of you – and that's the crucial point – are happy to try new things. If they don't harm or hurt anyone, there's no reason not to experiment. It's important, though, to go at a pace that suits you both, and for you each to consent and feel free to say that a particular toy or item isn't for you, so make sure you keep talking things through. But it's always good to try out something new if you both find it exciting.

On the subject of vibrators, the reality is that millions of women, either those who are single or those in relationships, use them regularly on their own for a rewarding sexual experience. Some older people – especially those brought up in a more restrictive sexual age or in more repressed families– can be uncomfortable about the morality of this, or they do it and then feel guilty about it, but most 20-something women wouldn't give it a second thought!

The world has changed a lot in the last few decades. On balance, the younger generation is probably much more well-adjusted to all things sexual and experimental. In any case, whatever people – including you – decide to do in the privacy of their own homes is nothing to do with anyone but themselves.

The Smart Woman's Guide to the Menopause

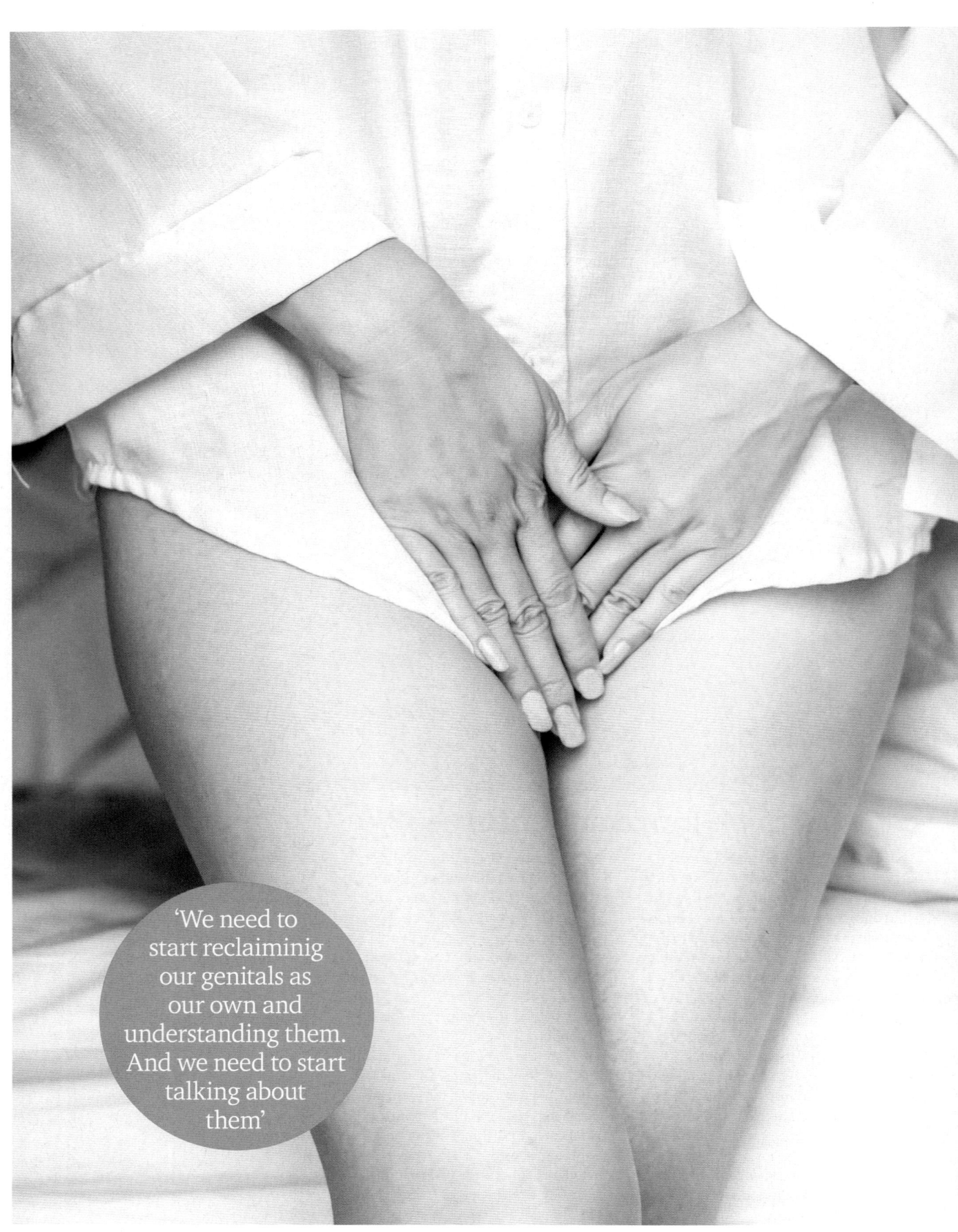

'We need to start reclaiminig our genitals as our own and understanding them. And we need to start talking about them'

EXPERIENCE

Me and my menopausal *vagina*

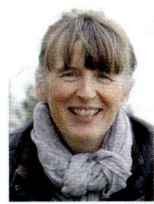

For many women, vaginal dryness in menopause can be relatively minor. For Jane Lewis, it was much worse. In an excerpt from her frank, personal book, she shares how vaginal atrophy changed her life…

Vagina. There, I've said it. Let's get the meet-and-greet out the way and get stuck right in, so to speak.

Ladies, before we begin, I think it's important to set a few things straight. We do not have 'front bottoms' or 'foofs', 'lady gardens', or 'minis'. Nor do we have 'clunges' or 'lady bits', 'fannies' or 'down theres'. No – we have vaginas and vulvas.

For too long, we have failed to really accept our vaginas, adopting instead the out-of-sight-out-of-mind mentality that has led to a culture of secrecy and shame. Unlike our male counterparts, our genitals are hidden within us, and that can often mean our suffering is, too.

We have been made to think that our vaginas and vulvas are something to be ashamed of, or that need to be groomed and pruned or plucked and shaved for another's benefit. We pluck turkeys, groom dogs and prune hedges; we need to start reclaiming our genitals as our own and understanding them. And we need to start talking about our vulvas and vaginas as they start to age: what to expect, what to do and who to see.

Society has somehow sanitised the menopausal woman; hot flushes and hysteria are the 'funny' stereotype. Cartoons are made of a woman standing naked in front of a fridge to cool herself down, or of a husband tiptoeing carefully around his angry, hormonal wife – who, no doubt, has crazy, frizzy hair and bright-red cheeks. The menopausal woman is stereotypically hot, forgetful and a bit manic.

The Smart Woman's Guide to the Menopause **87**

But what happens when we cool the flushes or level the hormones and start to deal with some of the other devastating symptoms: the vaginal dryness, the burning vulva, the suicidal depression? Why doesn't that form part of the stock character that a menopausal woman is cast as? It is simply unacceptable that vaginal atrophy isn't part of our vocabulary as ageing women. Just because it is hidden, doesn't mean it should be kept secret.

First signs

I'm not quite sure of the exact moment when things went so drastically downhill, but I do remember one day being at the cinema and suddenly realising that I couldn't sit down. After only 20 minutes, I took myself to the back of the theatre and stood alone, swaying from side to side, trying to calm the burning. I haven't been able to sit through a film since.

Fast-forward seven years and I no longer work, have visited an incalculable number of medical health professionals, wept my way around almost every local park and had my vagina lasered like a *Star Wars* lightsabre. Though I'm now much better than I was, there's still a long road ahead.

Today, I feel like myself – or at least more like myself. This is pretty significant because, seven years ago, I couldn't imagine ever feeling like myself again. I've just come back from taking the dogs for a walk and was able to wear knickers and even trousers all the way round. This is a small miracle. Even though I'm now sitting on a heat pad, trying to soothe the dull ache in my vulva, the fact that I sat in a car and wore knickers and trousers and walked – all in one morning – I think deserves celebrating.

You see, the thing is, unless you have experienced vaginal atrophy (VA) yourself and understand just how debilitating it can be, it's difficult to really get across how it feels to live with it every day.

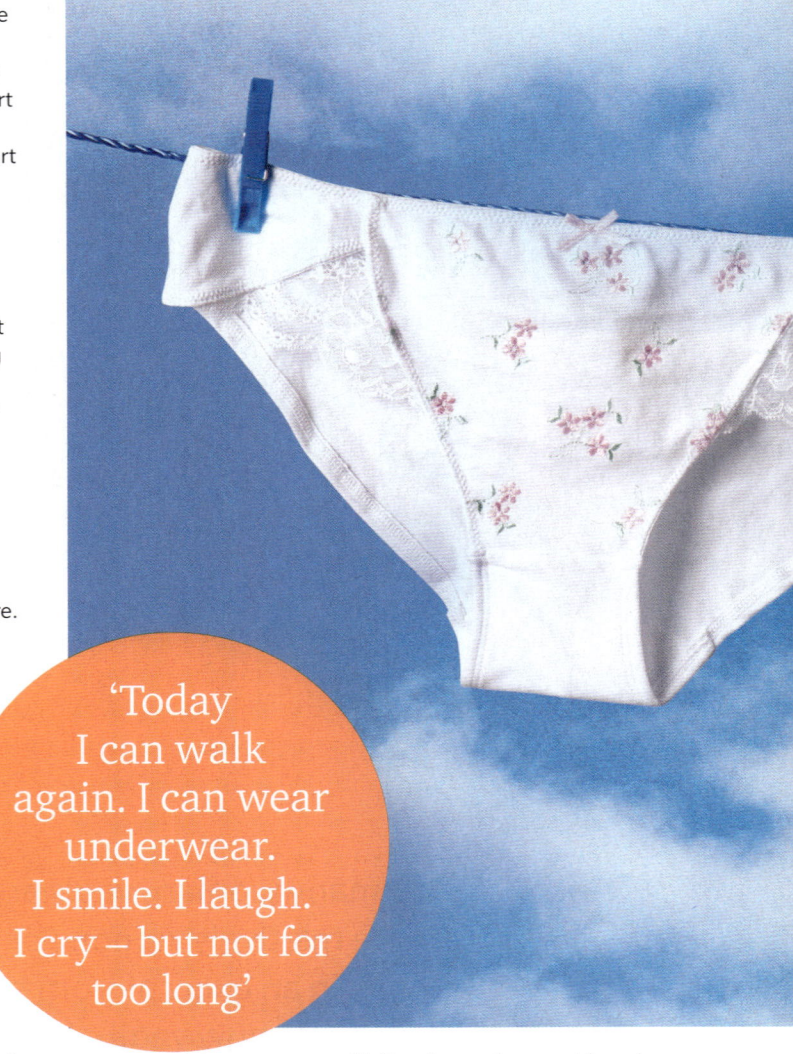

'Today I can walk again. I can wear underwear. I smile. I laugh. I cry – but not for too long'

A big decision

During the darkest days of my vaginal atrophy, I couldn't see the wood for the trees. I felt like I had literally tried everything to soothe the pain: homeopathy, moisturisers, yoga, meditation, hypnotherapy. I found nothing that helped. The only pleasure in my day came from the thought of bedtime, when I knew there might be a few stolen moments when my pain would cease.

For a while, I had heard from others about HRT and how it had helped them. But, for years, this was just background noise – I knew it was there, but it had nothing to say.

HRT is dangerous, I thought. *Everyone knows that. Why on earth would I take a drug that could give me breast cancer? Or poison my body with chemicals? Or increase my chance of stroke or heart attack?* I was desperate, not deranged! But, once all your options have disappeared, you find that your morals start to disappear, too. And that's how I came to HRT: desperate.

HRT, they said, could help with menopausal symptoms, including hot flushes, mood swings, night sweats and vaginal atrophy. *Including vaginal atrophy?* Interesting. Although I still didn't like the thought of being on a drug for the rest of my life, I knew I couldn't go on as I was.

And so, with desperately low morale, I dragged myself to the GP and asked about my options. I felt like I had sold out or that I was asking for class-A drugs.

> ❝ Unless you have experienced VA, it's difficult to really get across how it feels to live with it

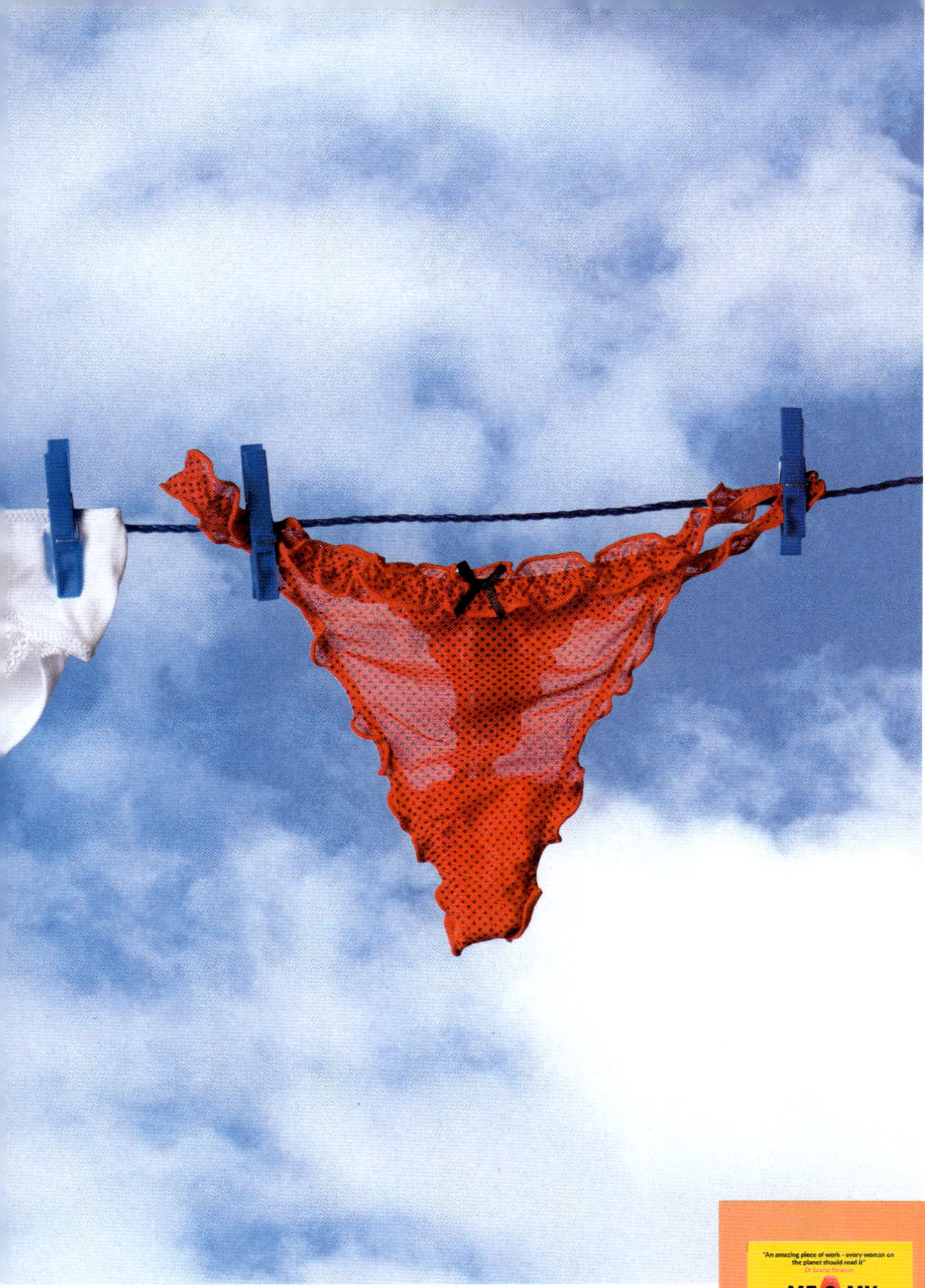

EXPERIENCE

Only 10 minutes later, I came out holding a prescription for HRT. One month later, my pubes started coming back. Two months later, my vulva started plumping back up. Three months later, I started coming back.

Brighter future

I'm aware of the possible side effects of taking HRT and whilst I wish on every star that I don't get them, I'm also pragmatic. Today I can walk again. I can wear underwear. I smile. I laugh. I cry – but not for too long. I can take my dogs across the fields. I can visit my daughters. I can cuddle my granddaughter on my lap. For me, that's worth it.

Whilst I've now come to accept that vaginal atrophy is a chronic condition that will stay with me forever and never be 'cured', there are definitely things we can be doing and using to go at least some way to offer more permanent relief. Try oestrogen if you can; visit your women's health physiotherapist; consider laser treatment; find products that suit you, and establish a strict routine that helps your VA. Be kind to yourself and talk to a counsellor – it may help.

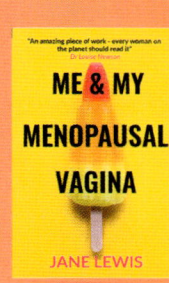

Me & My Menopausal Vagina: Living with Vaginal Atrophy (£6.88 PAL Books) by Jane Lewis is available at amazon.co.uk. For more information and support, visit Jane's website mymenopausalvagina.co.uk.

WHAT WORKS FOR ME

If you are new to VA or if you're chasing your tail about what to do, perhaps I can signpost you in some helpful directions…

✦ **OLIVE & BEE INTIMATE CREAM** (£17.99, 55ml, stressnomore.co.uk) This is a staple. I like that it doesn't contain any nasty chemicals and is easy to throw in my bag.

✦ **EMUAID** (£22.75, 0.5oz, amazon.co.uk) The antioxidants found in emu oil allow it to penetrate the skin deeply and ease the irritation from vaginal atrophy symptoms. Buy the best you can because some of them have added chemicals to bulk them out.

✦ **V MAGIC.** (£26.99, 59ml, stressnomore.co.uk) I use this in rotation with the first two external moisturisers above to ensure my skin doesn't become too sensitized to one product.

✦ **YES WB** (£5.99, 50ml, hollandandbarrett.com) This is a lubricant, but there's a range of products that are based in either water or oil, including a vaginal moisturiser that you insert into the vagina with an applicator. I use it in combination with the external moisturisers.

✦ **MEDITATION**
For me, walking with my dogs has always been my meditation, but I know of many women who would benefit from an app they could use on their way to work or when they're trying to sleep.

✦ **ORTHOPAEDIC MEMORY FOAM CHAIR SEAT CUSHION** (£8.99, physioroom.com) I take a memory foam seat cushion around with me and throw it down on every train, cinema or bench seat I sit on.

The Smart Woman's Guide to the Menopause

Coping with the 9 to 5

What would you do if hot flushes or brain fog began to affect your performance at work? Keep quiet? Leave? Not any more...

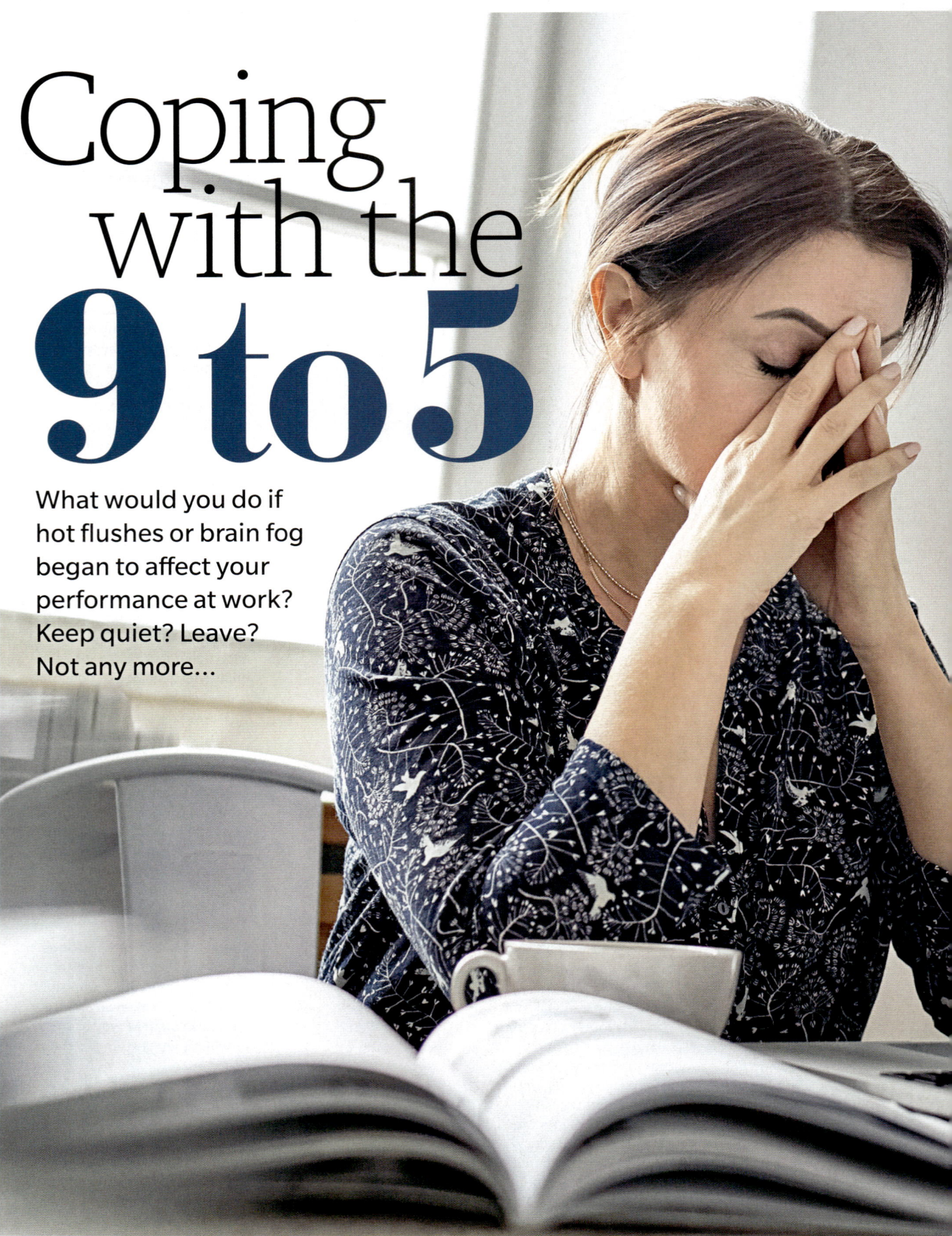

90 The Smart Woman's Guide to the Menopause

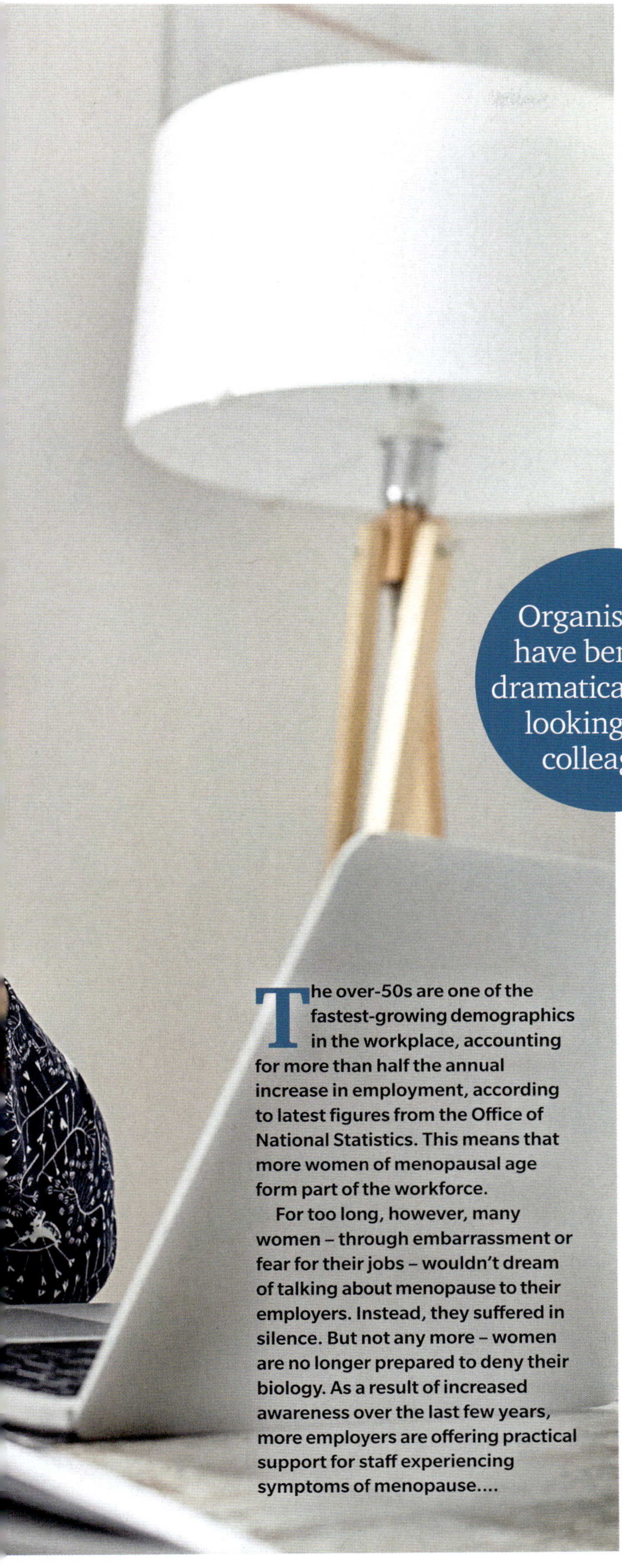

WORKPLACE

❝ Menopause support in the workplace is a win-win for everyone

Shifts in attitude

'More employers are starting to take menopause seriously,' says Deborah Garlick, director at Henpicked: Menopause in the Workplace. 'Organisations such as HSBC UK, Carnival UK, Sainsbury's, Northumbrian Water, Atos, Southeastern and NHS Trusts, as well as many universities and local councils, have all benefited dramatically from looking after the wellbeing of all their colleagues.'

This shift in attitude has come just at the right time for Lisa Williams, 47, an events and communications officer from Cumbria. 'Two years ago, I started to feel I couldn't cope with work,' she says. 'At the time, my team had changed and I got a new manager. I'd spent nearly 30 years working in high-pressure jobs and had always been a good performer. Suddenly, I was really struggling. I couldn't concentrate and my memory, which had always been my strong point, was terrible. At one point, I was worried I had dementia or Alzheimer's and I even googled some online tests. I'd also developed other symptoms – I had problems sleeping, dry skin, aching joints, night sweats, palpitations and hair loss.'

Lisa was signed off for a couple of months with work-related stress. 'When I returned to work, it was on a reduced basis, but I still felt overwhelmed,' she says. 'A colleague suggested it might be the menopause.'

Her GP suggested antidepressants, but Lisa refused, as she felt she wasn't depressed. 'I joined a menopause support Facebook group and was shocked to find that I had most of the symptoms,' says Lisa. 'So I went to see a private GP specialising in menopause, who prescribed HRT. This helped to alleviate some of my physical symptoms, but not the emotional and cognitive ones.

'I've tried three kinds of HRT, including the Mirena coil, which I had removed due to fibroids. I'm now waiting a few months to clear the HRT hormones from my system, so I can try a new type.'

Despite working in a male-dominated environment, Lisa's employers have been surprisingly understanding, giving her more time off and keeping her job open. Meanwhile, they have set up a working group to see how things could be improved for menopausal women.

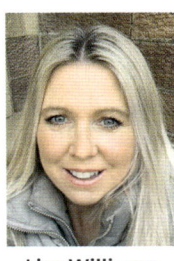
Lisa Williams

'I've been very vocal about my menopause because I think it's important to raise awareness so that women are offered the right support in the workplace,' says Lisa.

> Organisations have benefited dramatically from looking after colleagues

The over-50s are one of the fastest-growing demographics in the workplace, accounting for more than half the annual increase in employment, according to latest figures from the Office of National Statistics. This means that more women of menopausal age form part of the workforce.

For too long, however, many women – through embarrassment or fear for their jobs – wouldn't dream of talking about menopause to their employers. Instead, they suffered in silence. But not any more – women are no longer prepared to deny their biology. As a result of increased awareness over the last few years, more employers are offering practical support for staff experiencing symptoms of menopause....

The Smart Woman's Guide to the Menopause

Better training

'Menopause should be supported in the same way as any other health issue,' says Diane Danzebrink, psychotherapist, menopause expert and founder of Menopause Support, who launched the Make Menopause Matter Campaign in Parliament, in October 2018.

'When I launched the campaign, there were three aims,' says Diane. 'Firstly, to have mandatory menopause training for all GPs: most GPs receive very little if any menopause education during their training. Secondly, to raise awareness within the workplace, with all employers being given menopause guidelines for supporting women. Thirdly, to introduce menopause into schools in the Personal, Social, Health and Economic (PSHE) curriculum for all teenage girls and boys. I'm delighted to say that we've already achieved the third aim. Since last summer, all schools in England have now included menopause in the new curriculum.'

Changing the law

Diane is also working with cross-party MPs to push for legislation to bring in menopause policies in the workplace. 'Labour MP Paula Sherriff has been massively supportive, as has the Labour MP Carolyn Harris,' she says.

Conservative MP Rachel Maclean was the first to speak out about it in the House of Commons and has been campaigning for menopause support as a workplace issue. 'I became interested in this topic for the simple reason that it started affecting me,' says the MP. 'When I hit my 50s, my migraines intensified, but it took me a long time to discover the connection with menopause. Then I realised the need for this campaign.

'We now live in a society where women are working well beyond their 50s and 60s. Business needs talent right across the generations, and women of menopausal age are perfectly positioned to contribute positively. They are sometimes held back by adverse menopausal symptoms and through lack of education, understanding and basic treatment. So I'm on a mission to bring this issue higher up the agenda of government.'

Carolyn Harris agrees. 'You wouldn't dream of having a workplace where people weren't entitled to certain things because they were pregnant, and it's exactly the same for women in menopause,' she says. 'I firmly believe there should be legislation to make sure every workplace has a menopause policy.'

Far too many women going through perimenopause and menopause don't take promotion and either consider leaving or actually do leave, says Diane. 'But that has a financial impact on the individual and her family, and also on the organisation, as they lose a valuable member of the team and it will cost them quite significantly to replace and train someone. By implementing menopause support in the workplace, it's a win-win for everyone.'

> **"Business needs talent right across the generations**

> One in four women have considered leaving the workplace because of menopause, according to a 2016 study by Wellbeing of Women.

What employers are saying

◆ 'At Aviva, menopause is firmly on the agenda,' says HR director Laurence Beckett. 'We want to ensure that everyone going through menopause feels fully supported at work and is able to discuss with their line manager what would help. We are determined to stamp out any stigma around menopause and enable our employees to do their best work.'

◆ 'The symptoms of menopause can significantly differ from person to person and contribute to difficulties at work,' says Dr Richard Peters, chief medical officer at Network Rail. 'It was important for us to improve educational resources and raise awareness across the workforce to ensure those who are experiencing symptoms can feel supported whilst at work.'

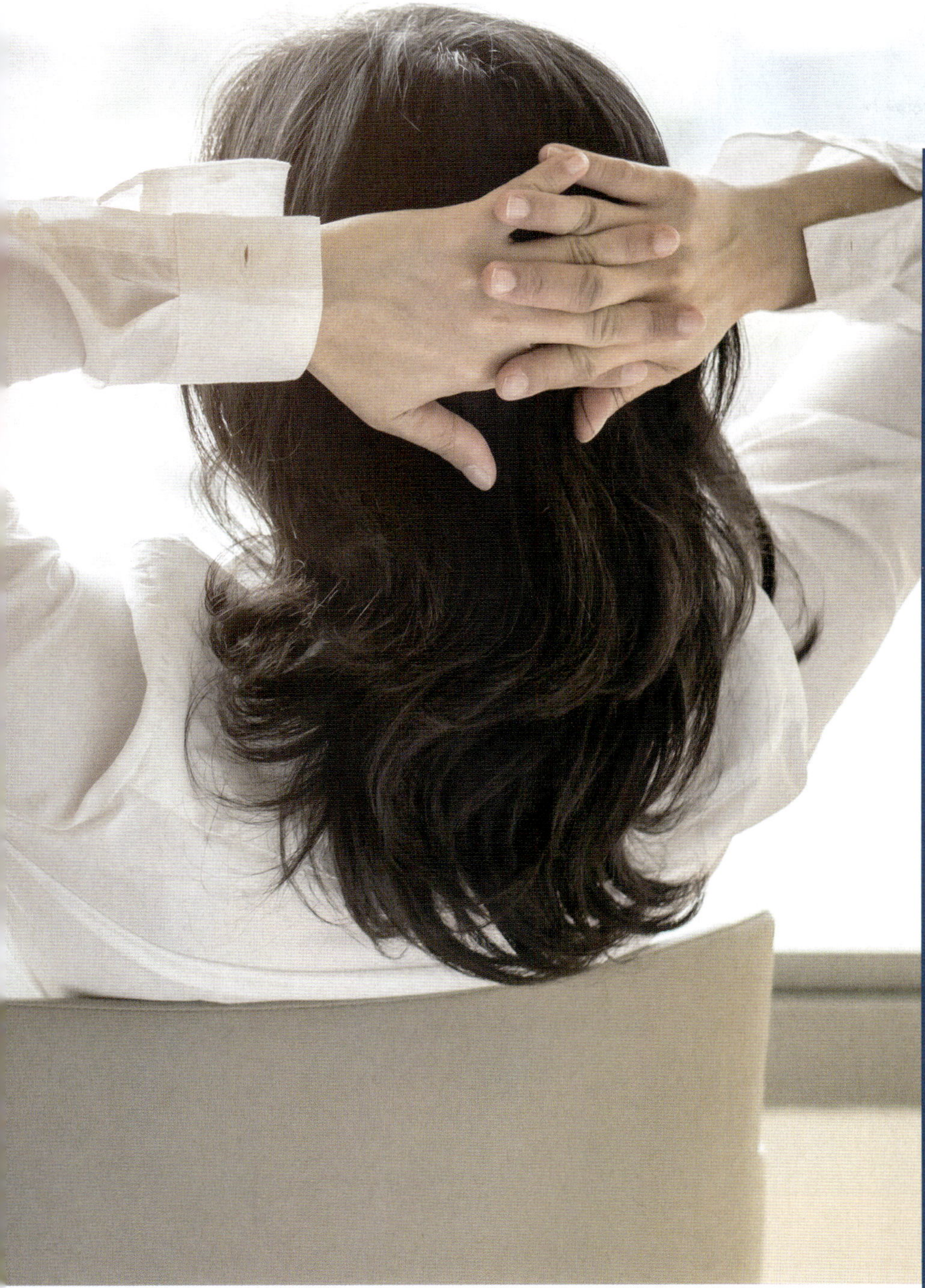

WORKPLACE

SIMPLE STEPS TO TAKE CONTROL

✦ Check if your company has a menopause spokesperson you can talk to. If not, book a meeting with your line manager. Try to overcome your embarrassment and remind yourself that your line manager is a professional, and that there is increasing awareness about menopause in the workplace.
✦ Book a time to talk, ideally in a private office.
✦ Prepare what you want to say: write a list of the symptoms you're struggling with and how they are affecting your work. For each, suggest a solution. This gives your manager or HR officer the opportunity to work out exactly what practical steps can be taken to help you.

FOR EXAMPLE:
✦ If hot flushes are a problem, you might want to move your desk near a window or ask to be provided with a fan. Check that you have adequate access to drinking water and a toilet.
✦ If some days you find it hard to concentrate, check if you can work in a quieter space or office.
✦ If you are having problems sleeping at night, leaving you too tired to think straight, ask if you can come in later some days.
✦ If you are feeling more anxious or stressed, suggest working at home some days.
✦ Plan a follow-up meeting to have an update.
✦ Think about setting up an informal support group at work. Check if there are other women going through the menopause and suggest meeting up one lunchtime a week.

CONCENTRATION DECLINE
In a 2019 survey that looked at 1,409 women experiencing menopause symptoms, 65% said they were less able to concentrate, 58% said they experienced more stress and 52% said they felt less patient with clients and colleagues. The report came from the Chartered Institute of Personnel and Development (CIPD).

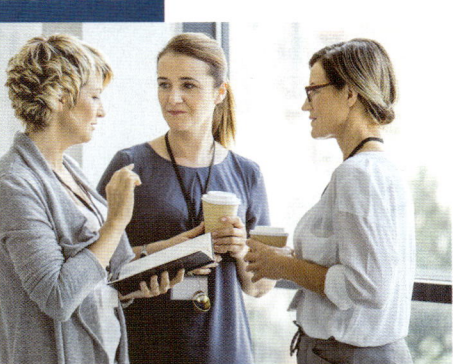

The Smart Woman's Guide to the Menopause

Finding a solution... *naturally*

When it comes to managing menopause, there are alternatives to medication

Movement can be medicine

A study of women aged 40-59 found that those who led sedentary lifestyles were likely to experience more severe menopausal symptoms. Walking, jogging and aerobic exercise will help maintain bone health – we lose 10% of bone mass in the first five years of menopause – and the feel-good endorphins released can lift us out of a slump and reduce anxiety. Try yoga, Pilates or swimming – or a combination of several types of exercise. By experimenting, you'll find what suits you best.

NATURAL REMEDIES

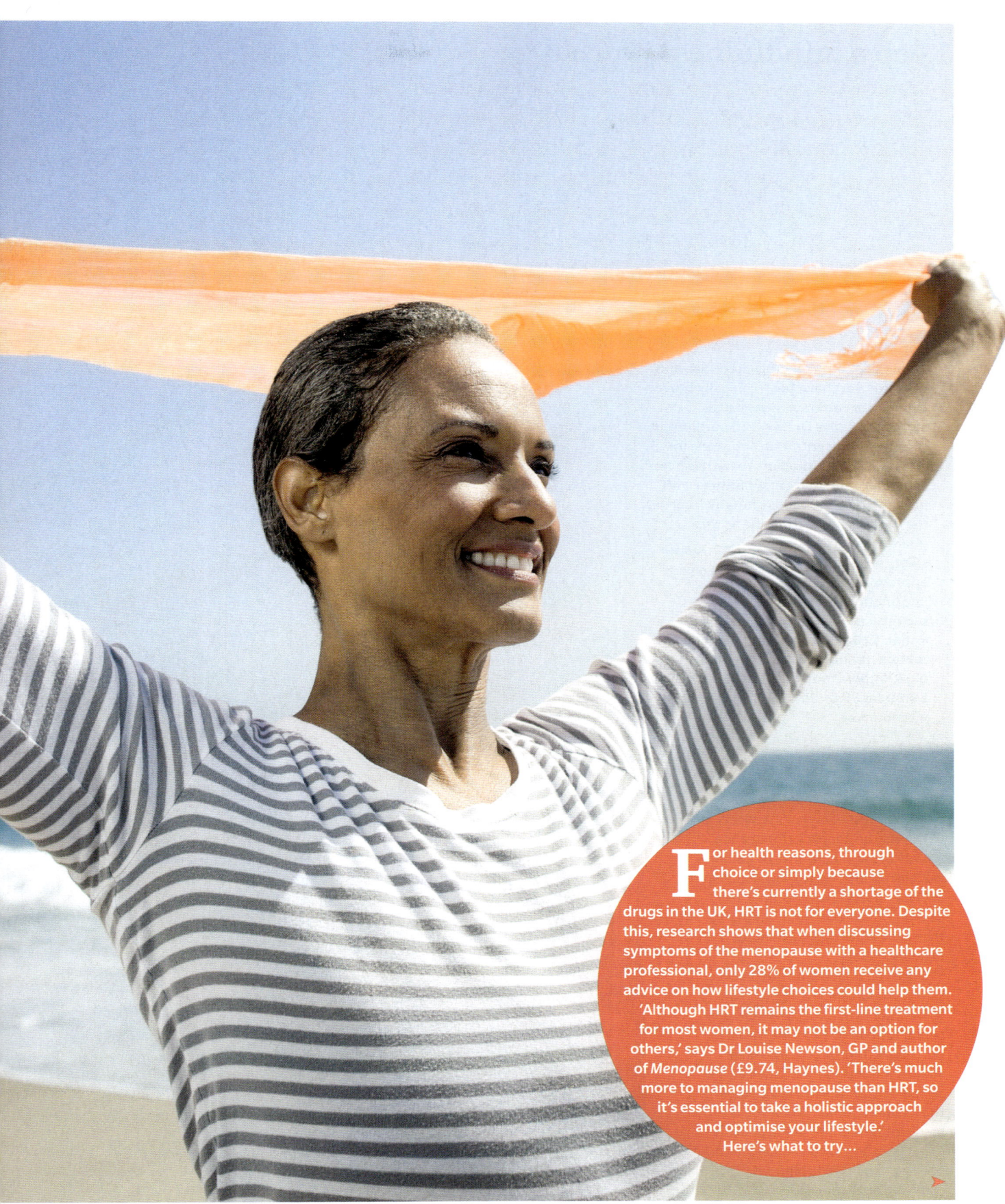

For health reasons, through choice or simply because there's currently a shortage of the drugs in the UK, HRT is not for everyone. Despite this, research shows that when discussing symptoms of the menopause with a healthcare professional, only 28% of women receive any advice on how lifestyle choices could help them. 'Although HRT remains the first-line treatment for most women, it may not be an option for others,' says Dr Louise Newson, GP and author of *Menopause* (£9.74, Haynes). 'There's much more to managing menopause than HRT, so it's essential to take a holistic approach and optimise your lifestyle.' Here's what to try…

The Smart Woman's Guide to the Menopause

Keep a mindfulness journal

Why not work your way through Goldie Hawn's *10 Mindful Minutes: A Journal* (Piatkus). Goldie has long had an interest in mindfulness, and her 'guided journal' offers insights, prompts and questions to get you thinking about your needs and help you feel calmer and happier. There are blank spaces for recording your thoughts and reflections, too.

Herbal helpers

'Remedies containing black cohosh and St John's wort have been clinically proven to alleviate common menopause symptoms,' says Dr David Edwards. 'And, if you find concentration and stressful situations hard, Rhodiola rosea has been shown to relieve stress symptoms with no side-effects. Choose one which carries the THR Certification Mark, as this guarantees quality, safety and includes approved dosage information.' **Menomood Menopause Mood Relief, £16.99 for 30 tablets, menoherb.co.uk; Rhodiola tablets, £9.90 for 30 tablets, vitano.co.uk.**

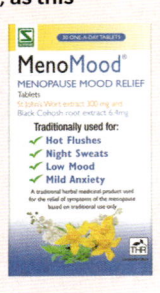

Lighten up with lavender

A great many women report feeling anxious during menopause, and this is due to oestrogen and progesterone fluctuations. 'Both hormones influence the production of serotonin, which is a mood-regulating transmitter,' explains Senior Menopause Specialist and Chair of the British Menopause Society, Kathy Abernethy. 'Alongside these emotional changes, physical symptoms, such as hot flushes and sleeplessness, can leave women feeling worn out and anxious.' Pharmaceutical-quality lavender oil has been shown to improve symptoms without the sedative side-effects of highly addictive anti-anxiety drugs like benzodiazepines. **Try Kalms Lavender One-A-Day Capsules, £7.16 for 14, kalmsrange.co.uk.** Feeling anxious? Turn to p110.

Hypno benefits

Hypnosis could sort out disrupted sleep, hot flushes and night sweats. 'It can also be beneficial for treating anxiety or low mood,' says Dr Caroline Houlihan-Burne, Clinical Hypnotherapist at The Princess Grace Hospital. In a session, you discuss your symptoms, then have around 15-25 minutes of hypnotherapy.

Once you understand the practice, self-hypnosis can be a helpful tool. 'Close your eyes, breathe deeply and count down from 10 to one on each out breath. Then repeat a positive suggestion in your mind, such as "I'll remain cool and calm all day",' says Dr Houlihan-Burne. 'When you're ready to come out of self-hypnosis, count from one to 10 and, on the count of 10, your eyes will open and you'll come out of the trance.'

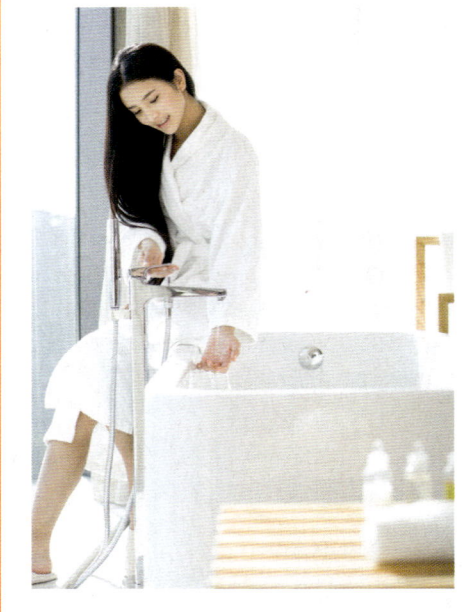

Have an Epsom salts bath

If anxiety is the problem, look to magnesium as the ideal boost. Nutritional therapist Hayley Netser says, 'It's wonderful for those who are a bit on edge, as it's very calming. You could have a small handful of almonds every day, as they're very rich in magnesium. Another way to boost your levels if you prefer not to take a supplement is to have an Epsom salts bath. Add about three cupfuls to the warm water, then relax in it for at least 20 minutes. It's well absorbed by the body and has a very calming effect.' **Epsom Salts, £5.99 for 1kg, westlabsalts.co.uk.**

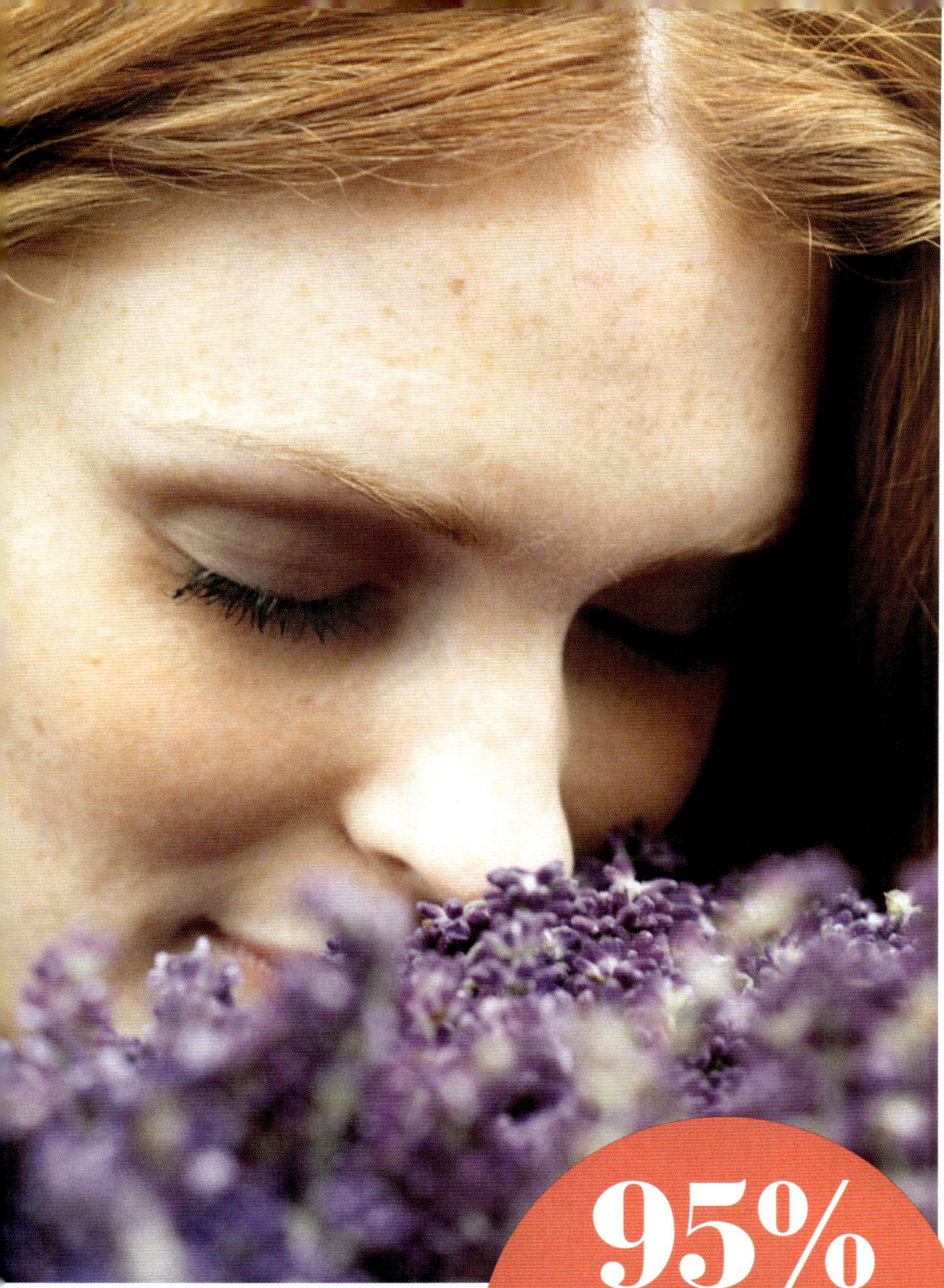

NATURAL REMEDIES

Symptom SOS

Women experience a wide range of symptoms when going through menopause. Here, we list the common physical and emotional effects you may be looking to ease.

- Hot flushes
- Night sweats
- Urinary symptoms
- Loss of sex drive
- Vaginal dryness
- Aches and pains
- Headaches and migraines
- Fatigue
- Constipation
- Irritable bowel syndrome
- Anxiety and panic attacks
- Mood swings
- Depression
- Brain fog and confusion

3 super supplements

- Hormone-free with purified pollen extract, **Femal**, from £26.20 for 30 tablets, femal.co.uk.
- Packed with ashwagandha, magnesium and green tea, **Botanical Menopause Complex** £26.50 for 60 capsules, wildnutrition.com.
- Plant-based Vitamin B, D and sage capsules, **Pukka Womankind Menopause**, £16.99 for 30 capsules, hollandandbarrett.com.

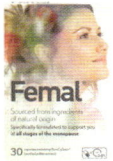 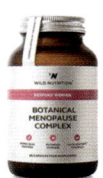 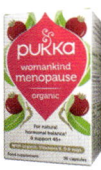

Make tomato juice your tipple

Researchers at Tokyo Medical University found that menopausal women who drank a 200ml glass of tomato juice twice a day for eight weeks not only almost halved their anxiety, hot flushes and irritability, but burned off more calories while at rest, too.

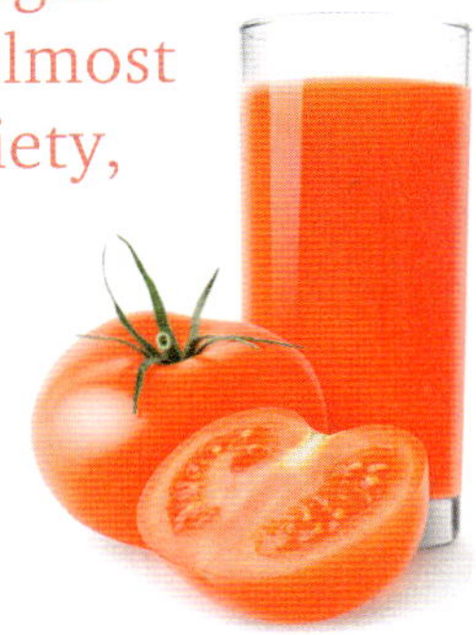

95% of women said they'd try alternative therapies before HRT due to worries about the health risks.*

Breathe yourself to sleep

Wakefulness at night is common during menopause. The 4-7-8 breathing technique is worth a try (but warn your partner about the 'whooshing'!). 'It's simple, requires no equipment and can be done anywhere,' says natural health practitioner Dr Andrew Weil, who pioneered it. Exhale completely through your mouth, making a 'whooshing' sound. Close your mouth and inhale through your nose for a count of four. Hold your breath for a count of seven, then whoosh the breath out through your mouth for a count of eight. Repeat the technique three more times.

CBD
your new best friend?

Products derived from cannabis plants are everywhere, but does this much-hyped ingredient live up to the claims?

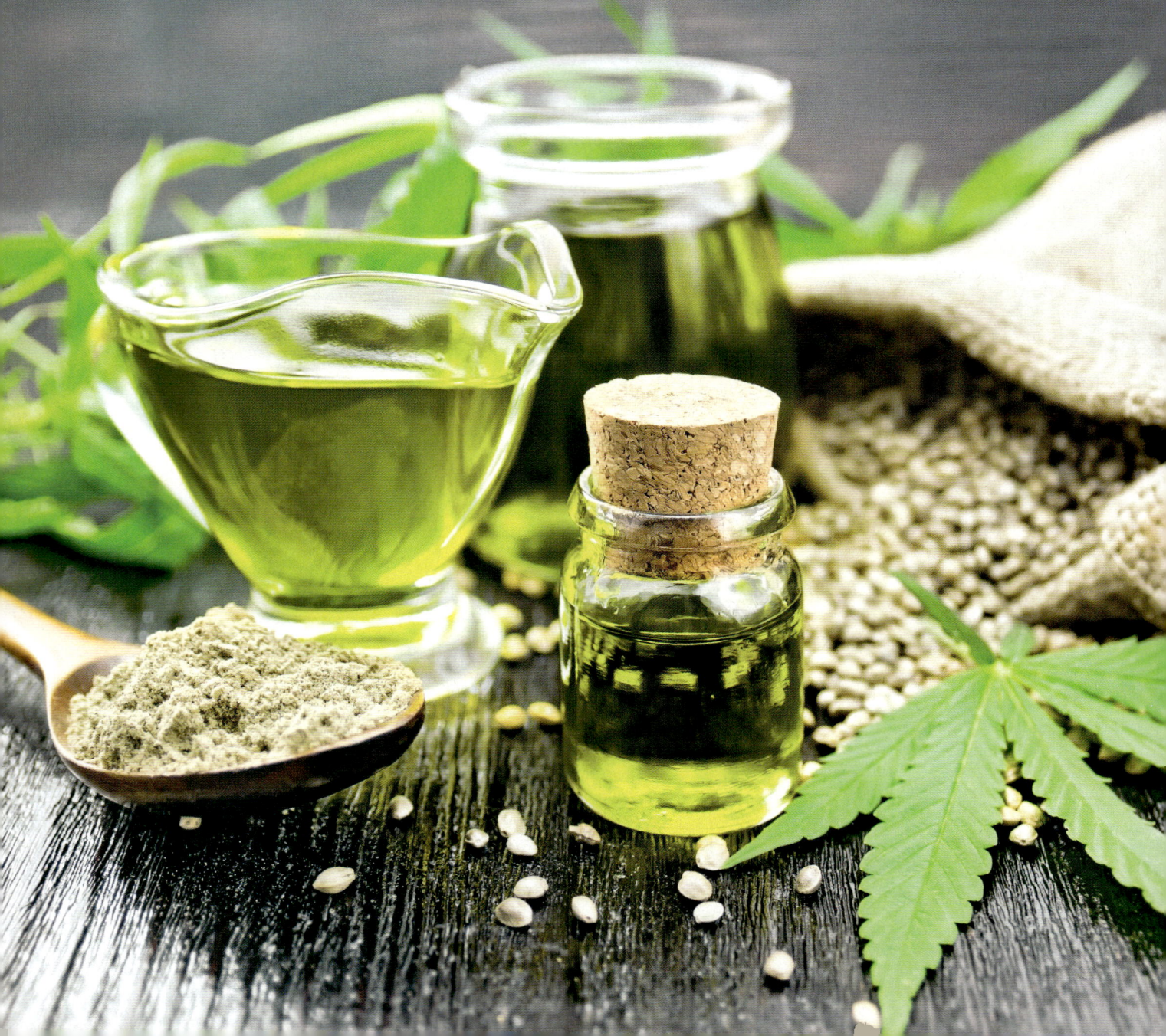

SELF-HELP

So you've hit mid-life. Whether you want to spark up your sex life, achieve a state of super Zen or have the best night's sleep of your life, cannabidiol (CBD) could be the answer. At least, that's the promise of a glut of new products, from infused chocolate and drinks to massage oils and creams.

There's been an explosion of CBD in the UK market, with companies extolling the virtues of products claiming to ease common menopausal conditions such as anxiety, insomnia and joint pain. Today, not only is CBD – usually in capsule form or oil in a bottle – available from health-food shops nationwide, but you can also ingest it in a range of snacks and even get it in sexual lubricants (it claims to improve arousal by boosting blood flow).

'CBD has become huge news off the back of some of the big medical cannabis stories that have hit headlines in recent years,' says Professor Mike Barnes, neurologist and author of *The Beginner's Guide To Medical Cannabis* (£7.65, Berrydales Publishing Ltd). 'Companies have suddenly seen the potential of selling CBD – a legal, non-stoning component of cannabis.'

Dr Yasmin Hurd, a neuroscientist and leading cannabis researcher at Mount Sinai Hospital in New York, says, 'The grassroots movement pushing for legalisation of medical cannabis in the US has probably triggered a swell of interest in cannabis products around the world.'

In the UK, a change in the law, allowing the prescription of medicines based on full cannabis for certain conditions, has also contributed to the growing interest in the plant's potential. But is CBD really the wonder molecule people say it is?

> **Companies have suddenly seen the potential of selling CBD**
> *Professor Mike Barnes*

Already on meds? Check with your GP before trying CBD.

What exactly is CBD?

CBD – or cannabidiol – is a molecule found in the resinous flower of the cannabis plant. 'CBD is one of many compounds called cannabinoids,' says Professor Barnes. 'It's closely related to another cannabinoid, tetrahydrocannabinol (THC), and it's THC that is the psychoactive "stoning" component of cannabis.

'CBD on its own doesn't get you high. Products containing less than 0.2 % of THC can be sold legally in the UK – full cannabis remains illegal to the public.'

What you'll find on the high street is usually CBD that's derived from hemp, a strain of the cannabis plant grown for its fibre content, which is naturally very low in THC. The hemp plant is different from the THC-containing cannabis plant people use to get high.

'Most of the products you can buy legally are from hemp, because it's easier to grow it outdoors,' says Professor Barnes. 'It's also easier to extract CBD from hemp without going above the 0.2 per cent of THC.'

Hemp-derived CBD is legal in the UK, US and throughout most of Europe.

What does science say?

'There is evidence that CBD does have medicinal benefits, but we still need more clinical trials to give us proof,' says Dr Hurd. Both CBD and THC are known to work in the body in a number of ways. Our bodies have something called the endocannabinoid system, which helps to regulate a range of processes, including mood, pain control and many more. If this system is either over- or underactive, the result can be various conditions, such as anxiety and pain disorders. THC and CBD help to modulate the endocannabinoid system, potentially easing or preventing these issues.

The other major benefit of CBD is that it's safe. 'No substance is completely risk-free, but the side effects of CBD are mild, including a dry mouth and increased appetite,' says Professor Barnes.

Is high-street CBD good enough?

'We know hemp-based CBD is less effective than the kind that's taken from "proper cannabis",' says Professor Barnes, who adds that it may still be worth trying hemp-based CBD supplements. 'The decent ones have lots of other helpful components, including essential fatty acids,' he says. Know what you're buying, though, he warns: 'Make sure the product is distinctly labelled as containing actual CBD. If you're using it to treat a condition, you should be looking for at least 10mg per ml. If you try one product and it doesn't help, don't give up – they can vary and it won't do any harm. If you're on other medication, tell your GP before you try CBD.'

The Smart Woman's Guide to the Menopause

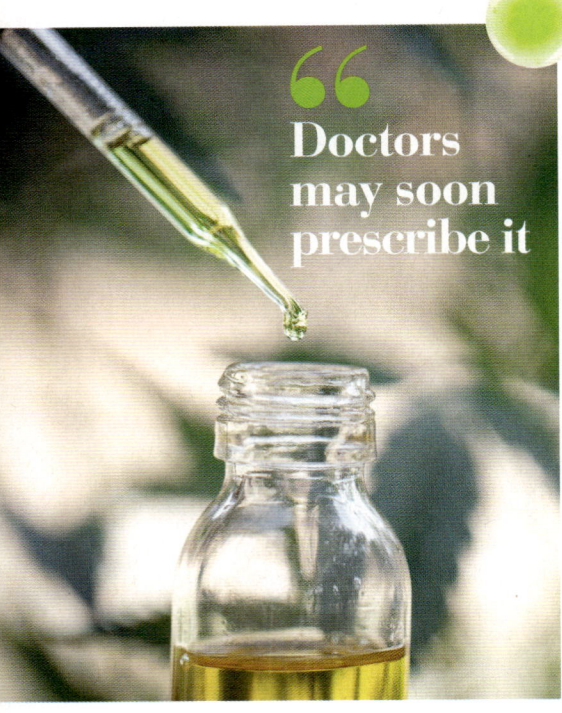

> **Doctors may soon prescribe it**

There is also the question of dosage. 'This is why CBD seems to help one person, but not another,' says Dr Hurd. 'It probably depends on individual metabolisms, plus any other medicine you're taking. That's why we really need more research to establish how much is needed for different conditions and different people.'

How about CBD moisturisers and other well-being products?

If you've found one you enjoy using, carry on – but don't be fooled into thinking that it will drastically change your life. 'There's no evidence any of these CBD products have solid beneficial effects,' says Dr Hurd.

The bottom line? If you have a serious pain condition that might be helped by medical cannabis, watch this space: a specialist doctor may soon be able to prescribe it to you.

Meanwhile, for many kinds of menopausal symptoms - pain, anxiety or insomnia – it may be worth giving some of the high-street CBD products a go. But read the label first to check it contains at least 10mg per ml – and remember, we all react differently.

WORTH TRYING...

The jury's still out on CBD but, if you're tempted, here's our round-up of products that promise a midlife pick-me-up

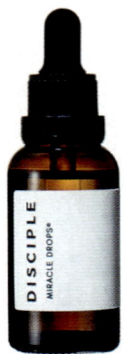

Disciple Miracle Drops 2.5% CBD, 250mg, £30, cultbeauty.co.uk
Apply to skin to soothe inflamed breakouts or add a drop to your coffee for a calming effect.

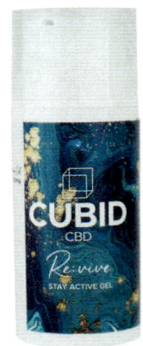

Cubid CBD Re:vive Stay Active Gel, 66%, 100ml, £55, cubidcbd.com
The CBD in this cooling gel is said to soothe post-workout aches and pains.

Healthspan Super Strength CBD Oil, £59.95 for 60 15mg capsules, healthspan.co.uk
Our tester tried them for a couple of nights and slept for longer.

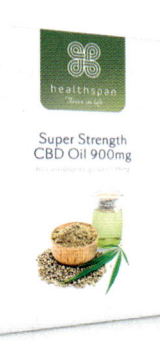

Westlab Mindful Bath Salts, £5.99, boots.com
You swirl these CBD-infused Epsom and Himalayan salts into your tub for bath-time bliss.

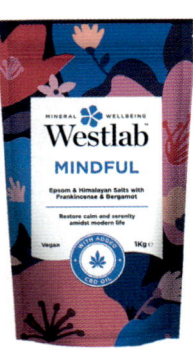

Green Stem CBD Bath Bomb, 100mg, £15, greenstemcbd.com
Scientists may not yet be convinced – but the lavender aroma is so relaxing.

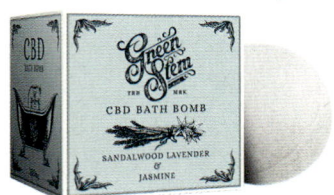

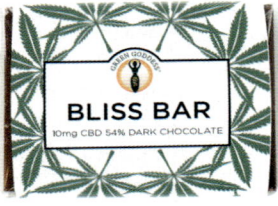

Green Goddess Bliss Bar 10mg CBD 54% Dark Chocolate, 50g, £3.99, greengoddesswellness.com
Delicious, but you'd need the whole bar!

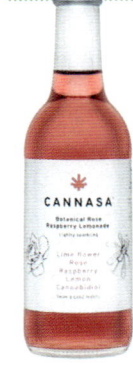

Cannasa Botanical Rose Raspberry Lemonade, 275ml, £2.99, cannasa.co.uk
A sparkling lemonade to lift your spirits, with no artificial ingredients.

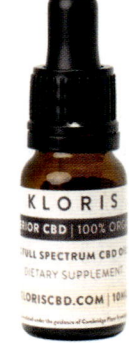

Kloris 500mg CBD Oil Drops, 10ml, £46, kloriscbd.com
Apply four to 10 drops under your tongue to alleviate anxiety, aid sleep and improve digestion.

IMPROVE YOUR FITNESS TODAY FOR A HEALTHIER, HAPPIER FUTURE

Packed full of expert advice and fitness plans, learn how to choose the right exercises, boost energy levels, break bad habits and understand nutrition

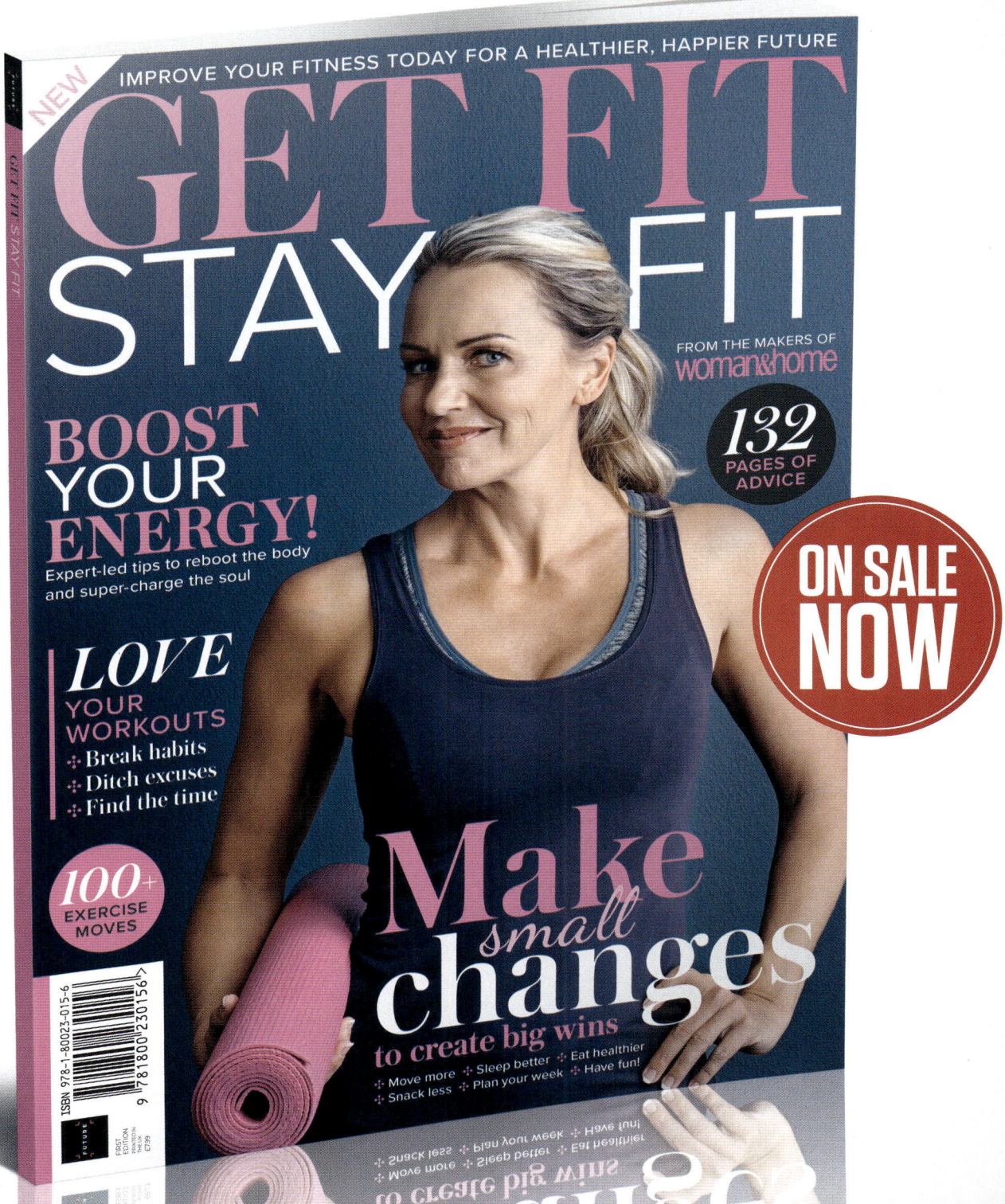

ON SALE NOW

Future

Ordering is easy. Go online at:
magazinesdirect.com
Or get it from selected supermarkets & newsagents

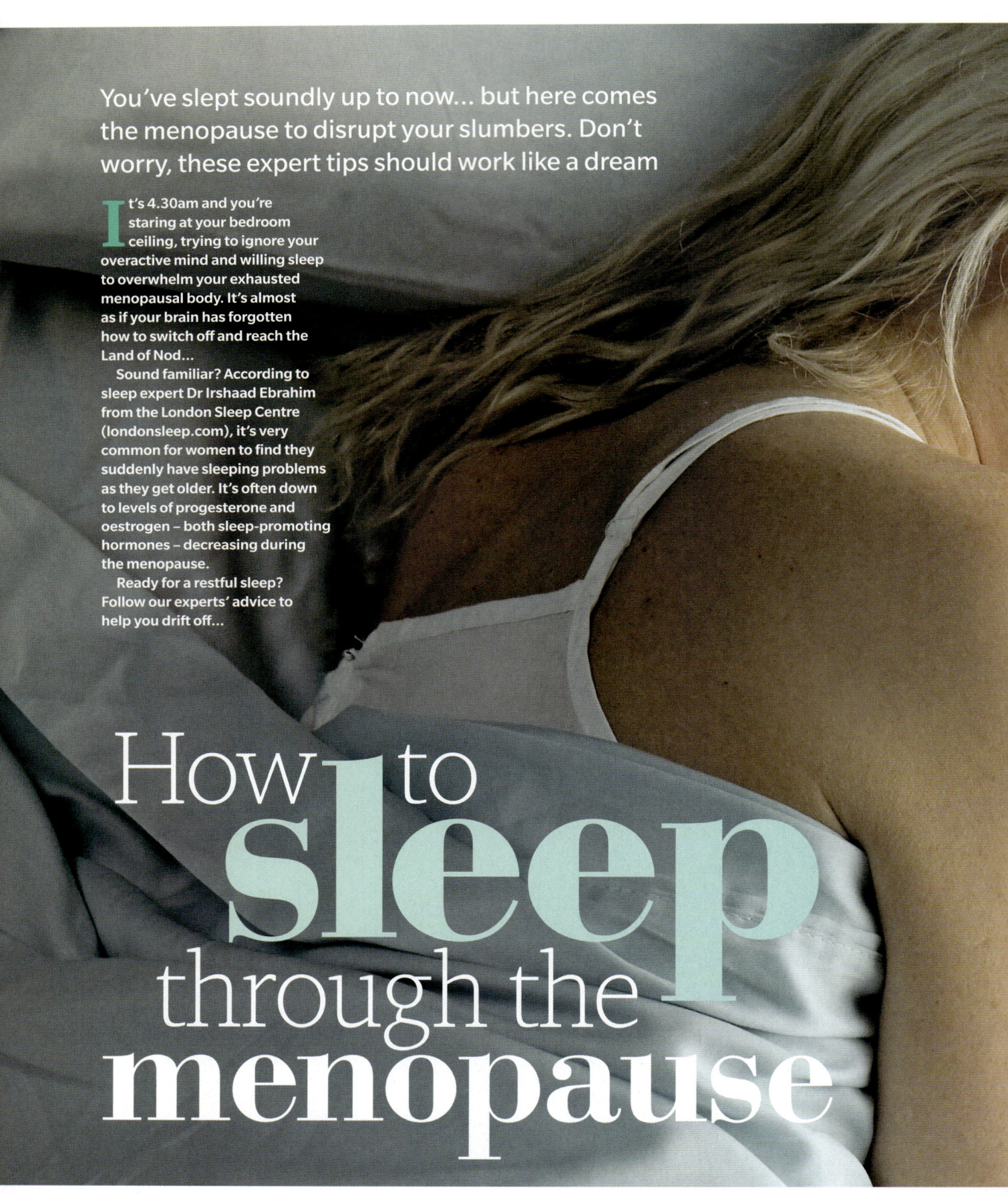

You've slept soundly up to now... but here comes the menopause to disrupt your slumbers. Don't worry, these expert tips should work like a dream

It's 4.30am and you're staring at your bedroom ceiling, trying to ignore your overactive mind and willing sleep to overwhelm your exhausted menopausal body. It's almost as if your brain has forgotten how to switch off and reach the Land of Nod...

Sound familiar? According to sleep expert Dr Irshaad Ebrahim from the London Sleep Centre (londonsleep.com), it's very common for women to find they suddenly have sleeping problems as they get older. It's often down to levels of progesterone and oestrogen – both sleep-promoting hormones – decreasing during the menopause.

Ready for a restful sleep? Follow our experts' advice to help you drift off...

How to sleep through the menopause

INSOMNIA

Changing habits

Even if you've always been a good sleeper in the past, chances are when you hit the menopause, restless nights will become the norm.

According to the National Sleep Foundation, 61% of postmenopausal women have reported insomnia symptoms. And those who do nod off may have poor sleep quality.

As well as our declining hormones, we also lose cells that make sleep-promoting substances, such as melatonin, and our brain volume shrinks, which makes falling asleep more difficult. What's more, we also get less stage 3 (slow-wave or deep) sleep, which is the most restful.

It's a common misconception that we need less sleep as we age. In fact, our sleep needs to remain constant throughout adulthood. If you don't get enough restorative shut-eye, you'll not only suffer from fatigue, but also potentially migraines, IBS, skin flare-ups and impaired immunity, explains Dr Nerina Ramlakhan, a sleep expert and ambassador for Benenox Overnight Recharge supplements.

It's a myth... That we need less sleep as we get older

Sleep is vital for our wellbeing

The Smart Woman's Guide to the Menopause

Tackling symptoms

Night sweats and increased anxiety during menopause can impact your slumber, but it's possible to overcome them and get a good night's sleep.

SYMPTOM
Hot flushes (aka night sweats)
These are the sudden feelings of intense heat that spread mainly through the face, neck and chest and are caused by changing hormone levels, affecting the body's internal thermostat. Some women get them at night and wake up dripping in sweat.

TACKLE IT
'A cooler brain switches on the circadian timer, this is part of the brain's pineal gland, which controls the sleep cycle,' explains sleep expert Dr Nina Ramlakhan. Keep your room well ventilated and between 16-19C, and sleep in cotton nightwear and sheets. You could also try these clever tips:
✦ Have a tepid shower or bath before bed. Don't use cold water, which will make your temperature rise.
✦ Soak your socks. Your body heat will cause the water to evaporate, lowering your temperature.
✦ Fill your hot-water bottle with cold water, chill in the freezer, wrap in a pillowcase and take to bed.

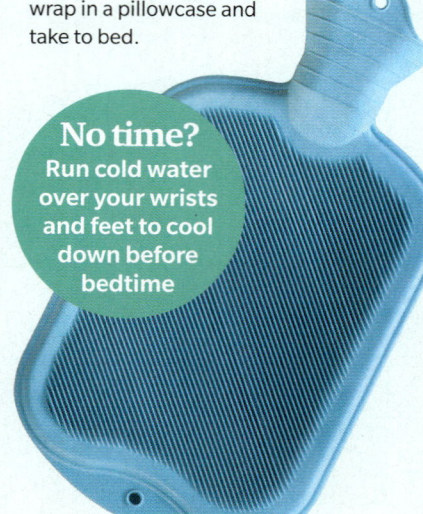

No time? Run cold water over your wrists and feet to cool down before bedtime

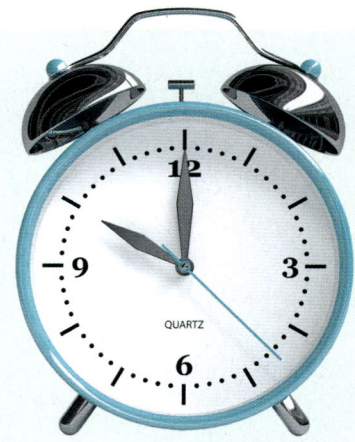

SYMPTOM
Anxiety
Hormonal changes, life stresses and worries about your changing body can all lead to anxiety at this time.
'Problems can seem heightened when we go to bed, and when we wake at night,' explains Dr Ramlakhan. 'From an evolutionary point of view and with the physiology of human nature, we drop our guard in the hours before sleep, which can make us more vulnerable to stress and concerns.'

TACKLE IT
'Most people wake up between 2am and 4am and struggle to get back to sleep due to stress and worries manifesting themselves,' explains Dr Ramlakhan.
Try acceptance and commitment therapy. This works for those of you who can't get to sleep or those who wake up in the middle of the night. It's all about accepting and acknowledging the negative thoughts that go through your mind when you can't sleep, instead of battling with them and trying to block them out, which can be exhausting.
'Learn to stand back from the thoughts you have and see them for what they are – just thoughts,' explains Dr Guy Meadows, clinical director at The Sleep School (thesleepschool.org). 'Don't push a thought away,' he adds. 'This can create more tension, which will keep you awake. Instead, just say to yourself, "Oh, there's that anxious thought again". By objectifying the thought, we can step outside of it.'

Avoid drinking... Caffeine just before bedtime so you don't need to get up in the night

SYMPTOM
Night-time incontinence
Pelvic-floor muscles may weaken with age, and reduced levels of oestrogen can cause the lining of the urethra to thin, so you may be at a greater risk of incontinence.
Stress incontinence is leakage of urine with exertion, such as from coughing, laughing or sneezing; urge incontinence is caused by overactive or irritated bladder muscles. The most common symptom is a frequent and sudden urge to urinate, with occasional leakage. You may need the loo several times a night, disrupting your sleep cycle.

WHY NOT TRY
✦ Kegel exercises to strengthen your pelvic-floor muscles.
✦ Cutting back on drinking caffeine and alcohol, which can fill your bladder quickly.
✦ Speaking to your doctor about bladder-calming treatments to help.

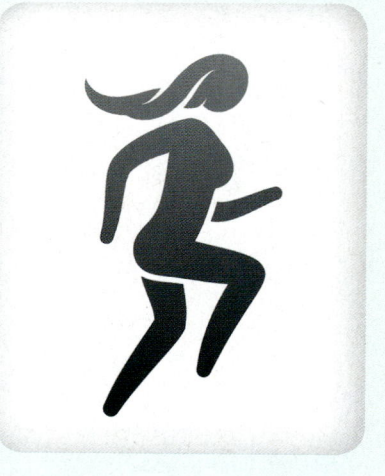

INSOMNIA

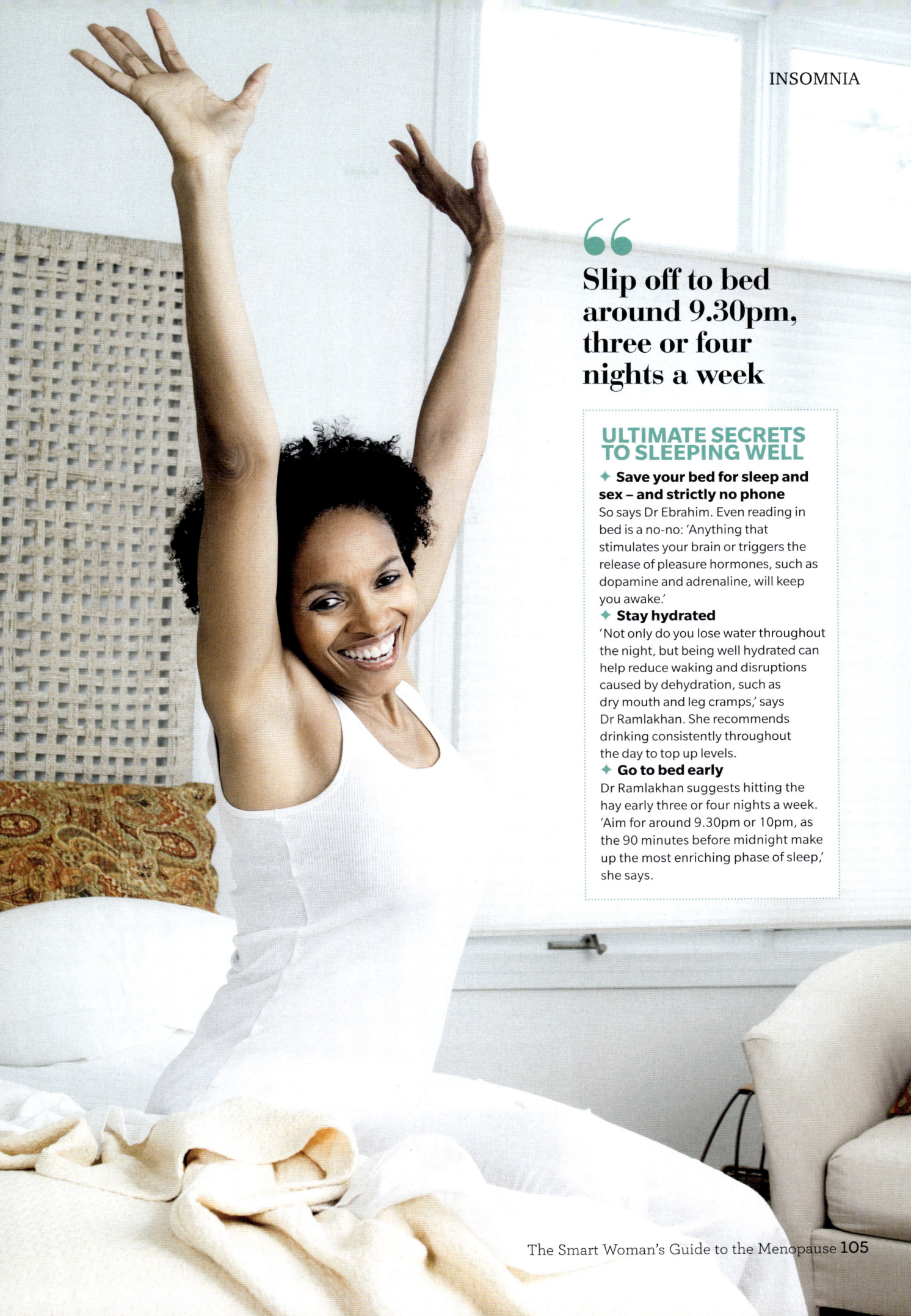

> Slip off to bed around 9.30pm, three or four nights a week

ULTIMATE SECRETS TO SLEEPING WELL

✦ **Save your bed for sleep and sex – and strictly no phone**
So says Dr Ebrahim. Even reading in bed is a no-no: 'Anything that stimulates your brain or triggers the release of pleasure hormones, such as dopamine and adrenaline, will keep you awake.'

✦ **Stay hydrated**
'Not only do you lose water throughout the night, but being well hydrated can help reduce waking and disruptions caused by dehydration, such as dry mouth and leg cramps,' says Dr Ramlakhan. She recommends drinking consistently throughout the day to top up levels.

✦ **Go to bed early**
Dr Ramlakhan suggests hitting the hay early three or four nights a week. 'Aim for around 9.30pm or 10pm, as the 90 minutes before midnight make up the most enriching phase of sleep,' she says.

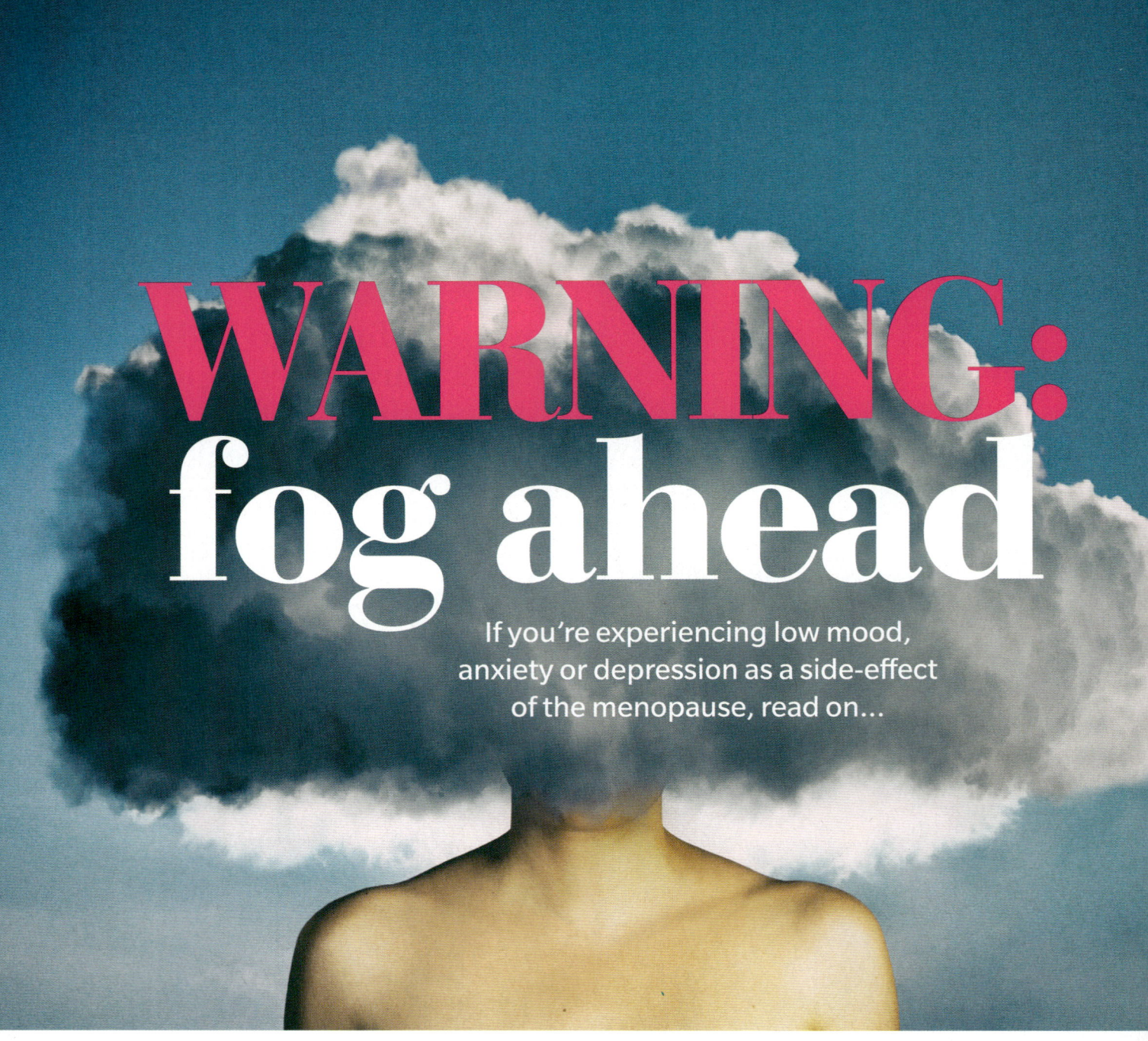

WARNING: fog ahead

If you're experiencing low mood, anxiety or depression as a side-effect of the menopause, read on…

When Laura Barton, 45, first started feeling anxious, she put it down to stress. With a busy family life and a responsible job as a deputy head in a large school, she assumed her lifestyle was to blame. 'I'd always been a naturally upbeat, energetic, glass-half-full type, but now I just felt gloomy, irritable and flat. Everything wound me up, I found it hard to concentrate and I'd often burst into tears for no reason. Some days, I felt I was losing my mind.'

Laura made an appointment with her GP, and blood tests revealed that she was perimenopausal. Her doctor explained that, as with more than half of menopausal women, fluctuating hormones were causing her mood swings and anxiety.

Balancing act

'When progesterone and oestrogen are in balance, they work together to keep the body functioning smoothly,' explains Dr Mayoni Gooneratne, a specialist in women's health issues (drmayoni.co.uk). 'In perimenopause, progesterone levels start to fall more rapidly than oestrogen, and this leads to oestrogen dominance. 'Low progesterone levels can cause symptoms, such as bloating, menstrual irregularities, headaches, migraines, tender breasts, weight gain, anxiety, mood swings and depression.' 'One symptom of perimenopause is cognitive dysfunction,' says Dr Megan A. Arroll, psychologist and co-author of The Menopause Maze (£12.99, Singing Dragon). 'This can make it harder to concentrate – you feel like you have "brain fog" and there may be problems with your memory. Often, women aren't aware they're in perimenopause, so these symptoms can seem distressing, confusing and frightening.'

57% of women have reported mood changes**

Emotional mayhem

The drop in oestrogen levels during menopause can trigger depression and anxiety, or make existing symptoms worse, adds Dr Arroll. 'Oestrogen helps to increase and maintain the balance of

106 The Smart Woman's Guide to the Menopause

MENTAL WELLBEING

feel-good chemicals in the brain, and also acetylcholine, the neurotransmitter that enhances memory and alertness. So a dip in oestrogen can lead to mood swings, anxiety and even panic attacks.

Consult a menopause specialist

'If you're of perimenopausal or menopausal age and you start to experience changes in mood, it's important not to ignore symptoms,' says Kathy Abernethy, menopause specialist nurse and author of *Menopause: The One Stop Guide* (£9.99, Profile Books). 'A lot of women say they can't stop crying or feel angry and irritable. Others feel totally flat and that life is a drudge.'

Even just being told by a medic that your symptoms are in line with the hormonal changes happening in your body – and that you're not, in fact, going mad – can come as a tremendous relief.

This was certainly true for Laura. Her anxiety and low mood were a result of low progesterone, and she was prescribed a very low dose progesterone cream. 'I could see an improvement in my mood within weeks,' she says. 'It was so amazing to feel like my old self again.'

USEFUL SUPPLEMENTS

◆ **Black cohosh** helps regulate the balance of oestrogen and progesterone. TRY: *Holland & Barrett Menopause Mood Relief*, £17.99 for 30 tablets.

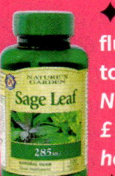

◆ **Sage** helps ease the hot flushes that can contribute to feelings of anxiety. TRY: *Nature's Garden Sage Leaf*, £17.99 for 100 capsules, hollandandbarrett.com.

◆ **B vitamins** support the nervous system. TRY: *Healthspan High Strength Vitamin B Complex*, £9.95 for 120 tablets, healthspan.co.uk.

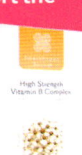

TACTICS TO HELP YOU STAY SANE

SEE YOUR GP

'Ask to see a doctor at your practice who specialises in women's health, as they will be more likely to have expertise in this area. If not, consider making an appointment at a clinic that specialises in women's health,' says Dr Mayoni. 'Your GP or clinic will arrange blood tests. Testing progesterone levels is best done on day 21 of your cycle, when this hormone is normally at a peak. Also, blood tests can give some indication of the ratio between oestrogen and progesterone.'

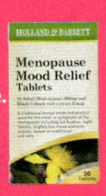

FIND A MENOPAUSE CLINIC

Ask for a GP referral, or you can go as a private patient. You will receive expert advice from doctors and specialist menopause nurses on all aspects of the menopause. For more information, visit thebms.org.uk/find-a-menopause-specialist.

TAKE STEPS TO IMPROVE YOUR DIET

◆ Avoid refined carbohydrates: instead, choose wholegrain pasta, bread, cereals and rice.
◆ Eat at least five portions of veg a day.
◆ Include healthy fats, found in olive oil, nuts and avocados.
◆ Eat omega-3 rich foods, including oily fish, chia seeds, flaxseeds and grass-fed meat.
◆ Try to eliminate sugary foods. These can cause insulin spikes that contribute to hormone imbalances.

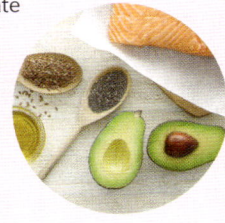

REDUCE STRESS

Too much cortisol, triggered by stress, blocks the action of progesterone, so try to reduce stress levels. Try mindfulness techniques like breathing therapies, meditation, yoga and hypnotherapy. Also try Headspace (free for iOS and Android).

TALKING THERAPIES

'These can provide you with coping strategies,' says Dr Arroll. 'Studies show that cognitive behaviour therapy (CBT)* can help to reduce the impact of menopausal symptoms with regard to sleep quality, daily life and overall mood.'

Ask your GP for a referral, or contact:
◆ The British Psychological Society (bps.org.uk).
◆ The British Association for Behavioural and Cognitive Psychotherapies (cbtregisteruk.com).
*Read more about CBT over the page.

With more women choosing to manage the menopause without medicine, we look at how cognitive behavioural therapy can help

Is therapy the answer?

There are around 1.5 million women in the UK dealing with menopausal symptoms at any one time, according to research by Women's Health Concern. And, increasingly, they are exploring drug-free ways to cope. Research has revealed that cognitive behavioural therapy, known as CBT, works well, too. If you've yet to learn about its benefits, here's the low-down.

LET'S TALK

Coping strategies

CBT is a well-established method for treating anxiety, depression and other mental and physical problems. It works by helping us to identify and change negative thought patterns that will then lead to positive changes in our feelings and behaviours, says The British CBT & Counselling Service.

Professor Myra S Hunter, clinical psychologist and expert in cognitive behavioural therapy for menopausal women, recommends it as a treatment.

'CBT helps women to understand the physical and mental factors that contribute to their experience of menopausal symptoms,' she says. 'There are strong links between hot flushes and anxiety and depression, and night sweats can cause sleep problems. CBT for menopausal symptoms targets all these areas and has been found to improve mood, sleep and quality of life, as well as helping women to handle hot flushes and uncomfortable night sweats,' she explains. The bonus is this: as well as CBT being available privately, you can access CBT treatment for free through the NHS' psychological therapies service, or ask your GP to refer you.

A course of CBT is typically five to 20 sessions with a therapist, lasting 30 minutes to an hour at a time.

'For women with troublesome symptoms, for those who have had breast cancer treatments, and can't, or don't, want to take medication, or for women wanting advice on how to deal with the menopause at work, it can be particularly helpful,' says Professor Hunter.

How to handle night sweats with CBT

Night sweats and broken sleep go hand in hand, so the key to managing wake-ups is to try to stay calm – and for this, cognitive behavioural strategies can be helpful. It's natural to feel anxious about sleeplessness, but with practise, falling back to sleep should get easier, says the Women's Health Concern.

✦ When you wake in a hot sweat, calmly get up and do what you need to cool down.
✦ Watch your thoughts while doing this – try not to engage with them and return the focus of your attention to your breathing.
✦ Once you have cooled off, get back into bed and practise 'paced breathing'.
✦ It's easier to deal with worrying thoughts during the day, so say to yourself, 'I'll deal with this tomorrow when I can think clearly', and return to your get-back-to sleep routine.

Calming those night-time worries

✦ **DON'T SAY...** 'I won't be able to function tomorrow'
DO SAY... 'I have managed before, so I know I can cope'
✦ **DON'T SAY...** 'I'll never get a decent night's sleep again'
DO SAY... 'This is tough at the moment but it will pass'
✦ **DON'T SAY...** 'I've got so much to do tomorrow!'
DO SAY... 'I can prioritise what I need to do and a bit of distraction will help me get on with things'

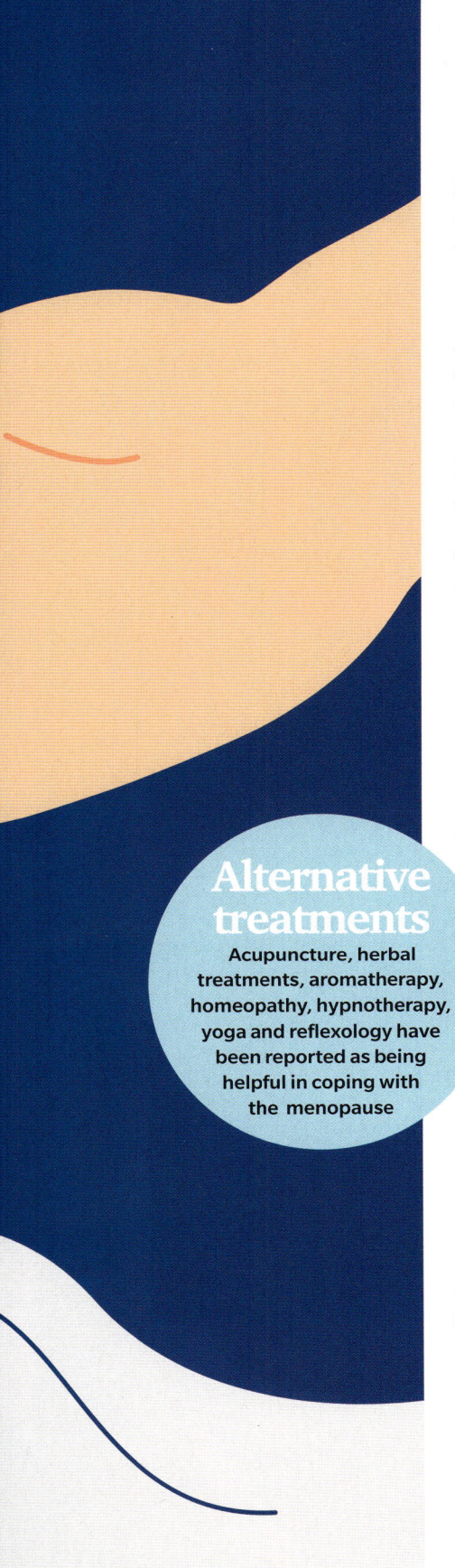

Alternative treatments
Acupuncture, herbal treatments, aromatherapy, homeopathy, hypnotherapy, yoga and reflexology have been reported as being helpful in coping with the menopause

Try this

'Paced breathing' is slow, even breathing from your stomach that increases lung capacity, bringing more oxygen into the body. Studies have shown that this technique helps with menopausal anxiety.
✦ Keep your chest and shoulders still. Push out your stomach as you breathe in, taking slow, deep breaths.
✦ Place one hand on your chest and the other on your stomach to help.
✦ The hand on your chest should stay fairly still and the hand on your stomach should rise and fall as you breathe.
✦ Relaxing the shoulders and focusing only on your breath lets you regain calm and control if you're having negative thoughts.

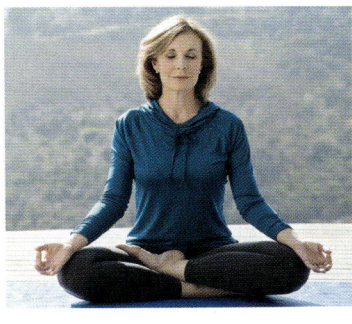

The Smart Woman's Guide to the Menopause

The age of anxiety

Many women become anxious during the menopause. Rebecca Frank looks at how to silence those dark voices…

Mention the menopause and most people think of hot flushes, irregular periods and maybe moodiness, but less familiar is the onset of anxiety which around half of us will experience during this time.

'People don't expect it,' says Sarah Rayner, co-author of *Making Friends with the Menopause* (£6.99, sarah-rayner.com). 'It hits women by surprise, and it hits them really badly.'

ANXIETY

Anxiety can manifest itself in different ways and we've all probably experienced it. The nerves we feel before an exam or fear in a threatening situation are a result of the anxiety response taking place in our nervous system. But for many women, those feelings don't pass, and the perceived threats become an everyday occurrence.

A study of 3,000 women showed half of women aged 40-55 had symptoms of anxiety, including feelings of nervousness or tension, irritability or irrational fear.

'Fluctuating levels of oestrogen and progesterone play a role, along with other factors, like work stress, family relationships and changing roles at work or at home,' says Kathy Abernathy, menopause specialist and author of Menopause: The One Stop Guide (kathyabernethy.com). 'And the symptoms themselves can lead to anxiety. Feelings like, "Is this normal? Can I cope? Am I able to work?" can be really alarming.'

Eye of the storm

Author Sarah Rayner started researching the link between menopause and anxiety after experiencing it first-hand.

'I'd had anxiety before, but as I approached 50 it escalated to unmanageable levels,' she says. 'I had physical symptoms including palpitations, rushes of panic, shaking hands and sweats. There were days when I was powerless to do anything.'

Sarah enrolled on an anxiety management programme and it was there that she began to understand her anxiety and to explore how hormonal fluctuations might exacerbate it.

'Of the 12 people on the course, nine of us were women of roughly the same age,' she says. 'As a writer this intrigued me, so I started researching it and ended up writing two books, one on anxiety and one on the menopause (with GP, Dr Patrick Fitzgerald).' Sarah believes that understanding the causes of anxiety so she could recognise the symptoms and think 'that's adrenaline' rather than 'what the hell's happening to me?' helped to de-escalate her panic.

Body changes

Changes to our body during midlife can also provoke feelings of anxiety. Weight seems to shift to the tummy and it's harder to lose. Muscle tone might change, skin becomes drier and it's common to experience a loss of libido and problems with sex. Hormonal changes may also play a role in the onset of eating disorders. Perimenopause is a time when hormones are shifting and experts say there needs to be more awareness of eating disorders among middle-aged women.

What's up? Hormonal changes may play a role in the onset of eating disorders in middle-aged women. A study in *BMC Medicine* showed that 3.6% are currently affected

Finding calm

'Recognising the symptoms of anxiety and that they won't last for ever helps stop it from escalating,' says Kathy. Calming activities, such as breathing and mindfulness exercises, will neutralise the anxiety hormones and improve sleep and try natural remedies to reduce anxiety, like lavender oil (try *Kalms Lavender One-A-Day £6.49, Boots*) and CBD oil (try *Dragonfly CBD Narrow-Spectrum Oil, £25, dragonflycbd.com*).

'I found yoga really helpful,' says Sarah. 'The combination of guided breathing and being with other people worked for me.' Sarah hosts a Facebook group, Making Friends with the Menopause, where around 4,400 women share experiences and support each other. 'We're all spinning many plates. One minute we're a career woman, the next a carer to a parent or parent to a teenager leaving home, and it can all feel too much,' she says.

Asking for help

If you feel like anxiety is stopping you from living life or affecting your decisions, don't hesitate to get help. 'Anxiety is anxiety's own best friend and you can only break that cycle by doing something about it,' says Sarah. 'Ask to see a GP with an interest in women's health and explain how you feel. Don't be ashamed to ask for help.'

'I couldn't trust my own judgement any more'

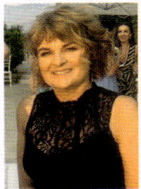

Midway through the menopause Karen Palmes, now 57, began to feel anxious. Now happily through the worst, she reveals what helped…

'I'd started feeling low in my mid 40s, a year or so prior to my symptoms starting, and had been taking St John's wort, which seemed to lift my mood. Then things started to escalate and along with the onset of hot flushes, I felt suddenly anxious and out of control of my emotions. I would be shouting one minute and crying the next, and didn't seem to be able judge situations or people's behaviour towards me in a rational way. I just couldn't trust my own judgement any more and I knew I needed to do something about it.

I talked to my GP, who took a blood test that showed my oestrogen levels had dropped considerably and quickly. It was a relief to know the reason for how I was feeling. We decided I should try a low-dosage HRT.

I noticed a huge difference within weeks. I felt calmer and on top of things again. The hot flushes also stopped so I was able to sleep better. I stayed on HRT for five years and when I came off it at 53, I was worried that my symptoms might recur, but thankfully they didn't.

Going on HRT was definitely the right thing for me, I couldn't have carried on like that!'

The Smart Woman's Guide to the Menopause

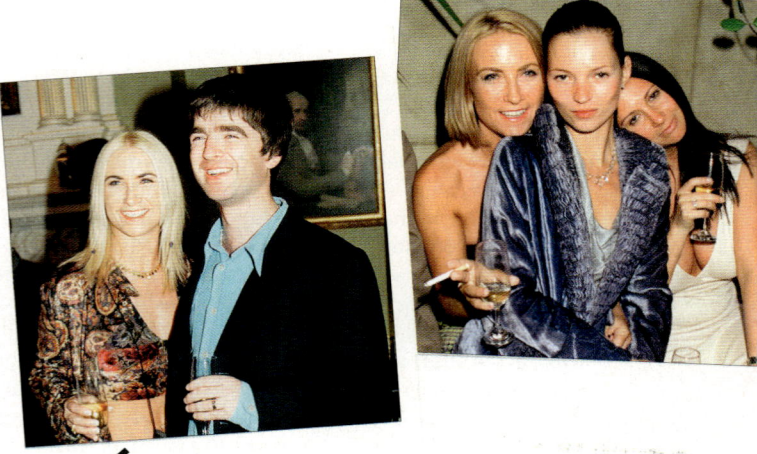
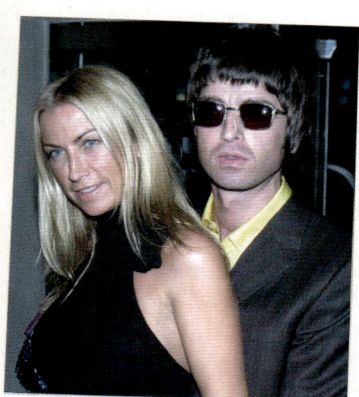

'I thought the 90s had caught up with me *but it was the MENOPAUSE!*'

Eight years ago, Meg Mathews – a well-known part of the Britpop music scene – noticed worrying symptoms. Here she explains what happened next…

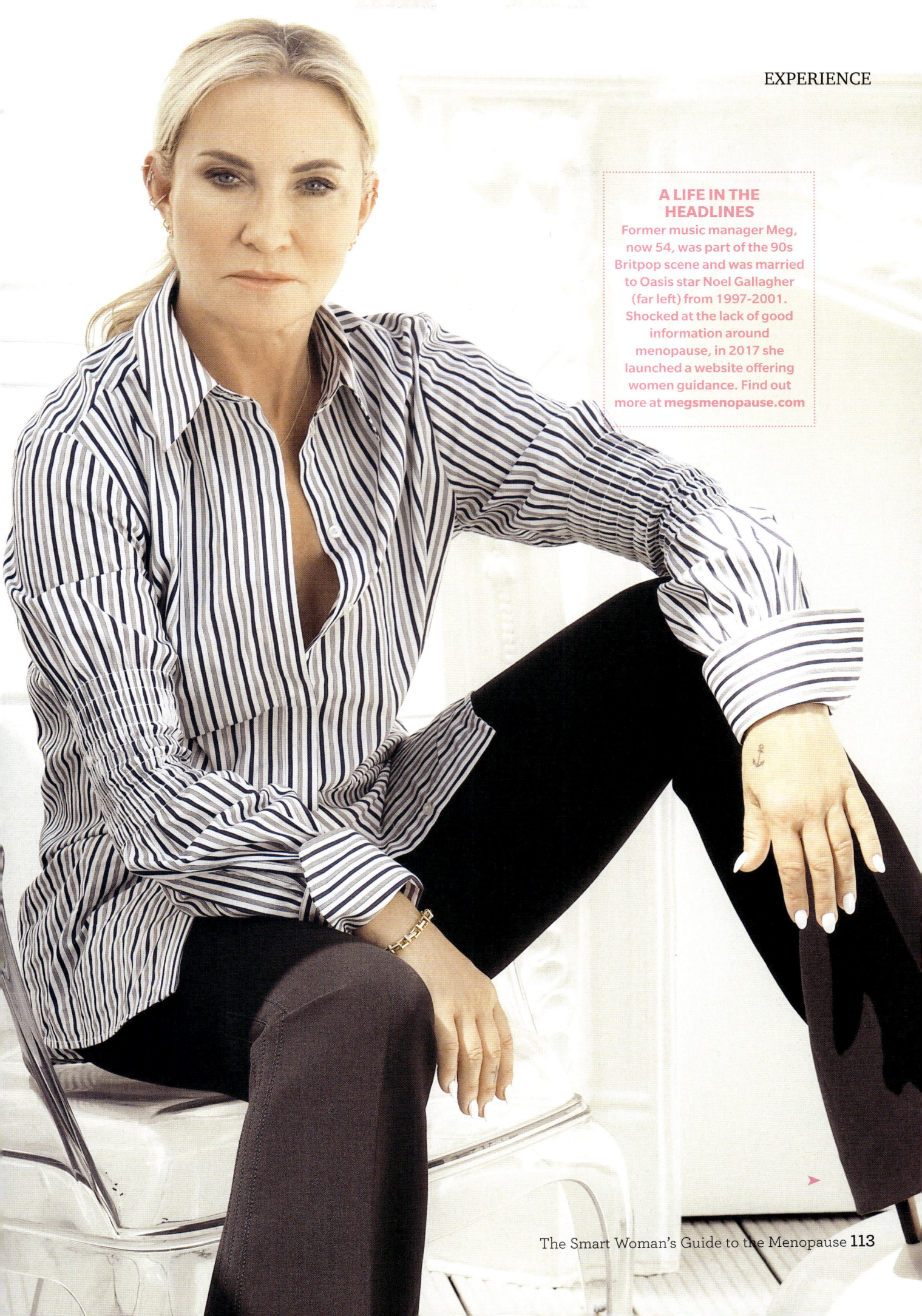

EXPERIENCE

A LIFE IN THE HEADLINES
Former music manager Meg, now 54, was part of the 90s Britpop scene and was married to Oasis star Noel Gallagher (far left) from 1997-2001. Shocked at the lack of good information around menopause, in 2017 she launched a website offering women guidance. Find out more at megsmenopause.com

The Smart Woman's Guide to the Menopause

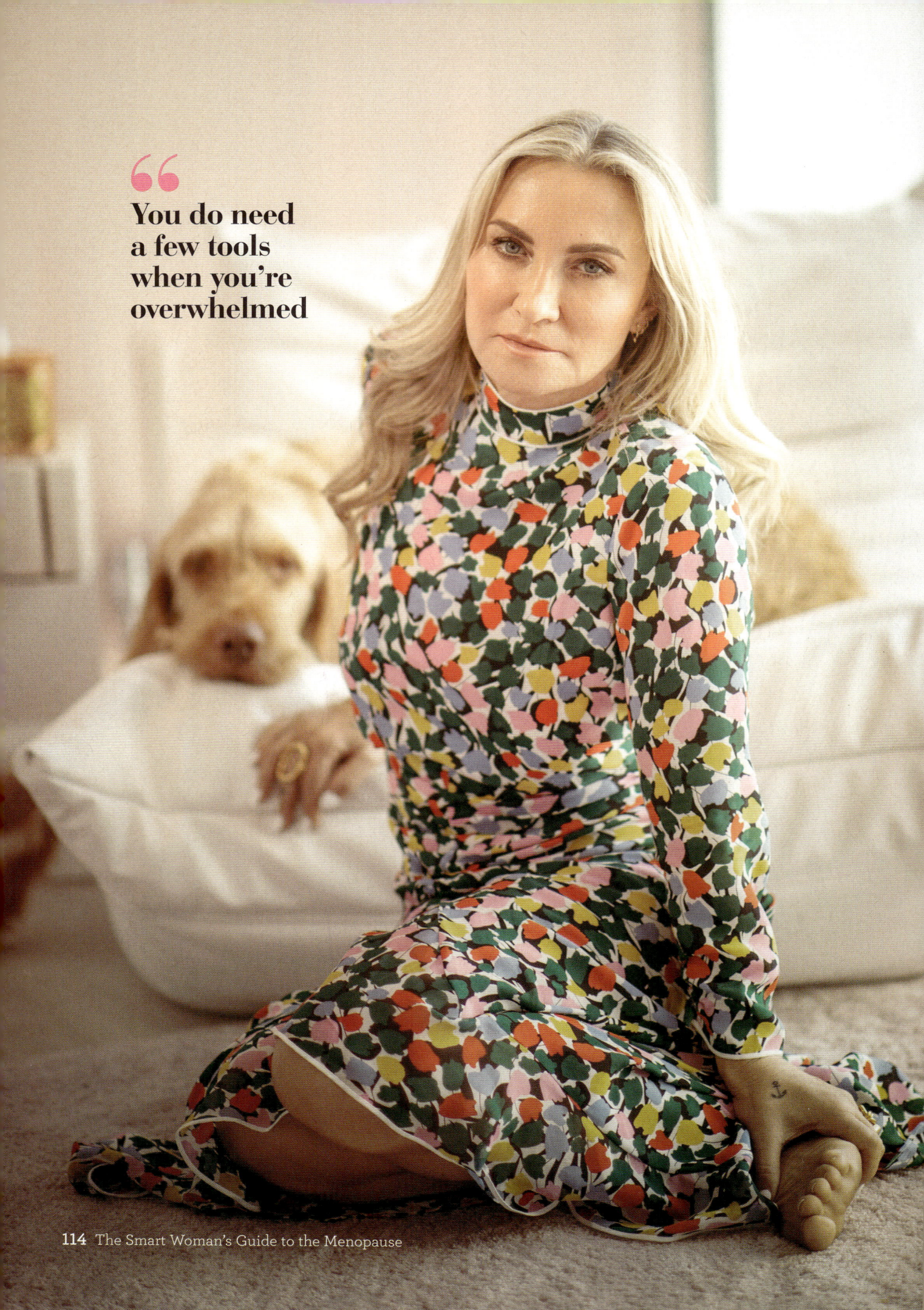

> You do need a few tools when you're overwhelmed

EXPERIENCE

Menopause took me to a new part of my life

When it first started I didn't know what was going on. I wasn't in a good space, I had a foggy brain, I couldn't sleep and I had the worst anxiety. I felt overwhelmed by life, my joints ached and I felt nauseous. Everything was why, why? Why couldn't I go to the gym? Why was there no information out there? All of a sudden, I had no energy and I thought I'd burned myself out. I thought my colourful years in the 90s had caught up with me. (My mum always said they would one day!)

We need to change the language

When I realised I was going through the menopause, it became important to me that women should understand sooner what's going on. I'd have liked to be able to read something and think 'that's me' and 'that's what I can do'.

Physically, I was back on track…

I had aching joints, which was very alien to me. But, once I started rubbing an oestrogen therapy gel on my inner thighs, I felt amazing. In four days, my night sweats had stopped, and within about a month I was practically back to normal. Oestrogen is a very powerful hormone, which I believe we need to replace.

But I needed more support

We women take on a lot, and we feel guilty if we focus on ourselves. We have to change all that. Don't be a martyr – share your feelings with your family. You need the support and you'll feel so much better. Tell your kids, 'I'm not feeling 100% today'. Then, when they see you crying at an advert, it will make sense. The more you put it out there, the more they will understand.

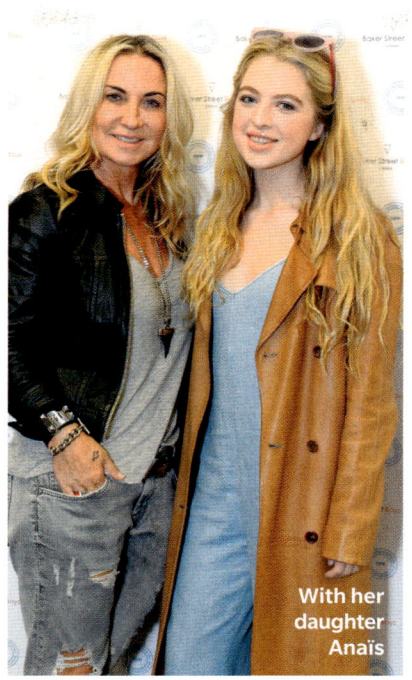

With her daughter Anaïs

There should be help for others

It's still taboo to be as outgoing as I am, especially in the workplace, but it should be employers' responsibility to support women through menopause. There should be something in place within HR, and I'm a real advocate of that. In fact, I want to work with the health minister to get this changed.

A large percentage of women going through the menopause are still working, and they shouldn't have to 'come out' about it. They should be able to work flexible hours; they need to be hydrated; they need to have a room they can go to – space where they can gather themselves and be able to take a little bit of time out.

My dream is to have Meg's Menopause meetings – a bit like Weight Watchers! I'd love women to be able to join a group, find support and talk to other women – and for them to say 'I'm going through this, too'.

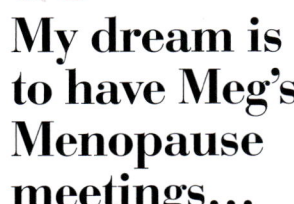

> My dream is to have Meg's Menopause meetings…

MEG'S GO-TO SOLUTIONS FOR MENOPAUSE SYMPTOMS

✦ HAIR LOSS
When I put hormones back in my body, it was like, 'Wow! Thank you!' – and my hair got thick again. I know some women can't take HRT, though. I do feel that it's important to change your shampoo and conditioner as your hair gets used to it.

✦ INTIMACY
It is pretty difficult at this age. Your libido isn't as high as it was, so you need to have a proper connection with somebody. Focus more on the desire and being intimate with that – holding hands, going to a movie or for a walk – old-fashioned courting.

✦ MENTAL HEALTH
My anxiety was so bad, I didn't leave my house for three months. CBD oil really helped me. You do need a few tools when you're feeling overwhelmed. I love oils, crystals, chakra sprays – anything I can breathe that makes me feel centred. And talk to people – tell someone when you're not OK.

✦ FLUSHES
When I feel hot or overwhelmed, I spritz on some **Rosey Rain Facial Cooling Spray (£15, 60ml, megsmenopause.com)** and really breathe. It helps me reconnect. Breathing helps whenever you feel a hot flush rising up. I breathe in for a count of five, hold for five, then breathe out for five. I call it 'the changing breath' and I do it a few times with my eyes closed. Find a quiet space if you're feeling anxious and do this – it's a really good one!

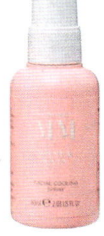

The Smart Woman's Guide to the Menopause

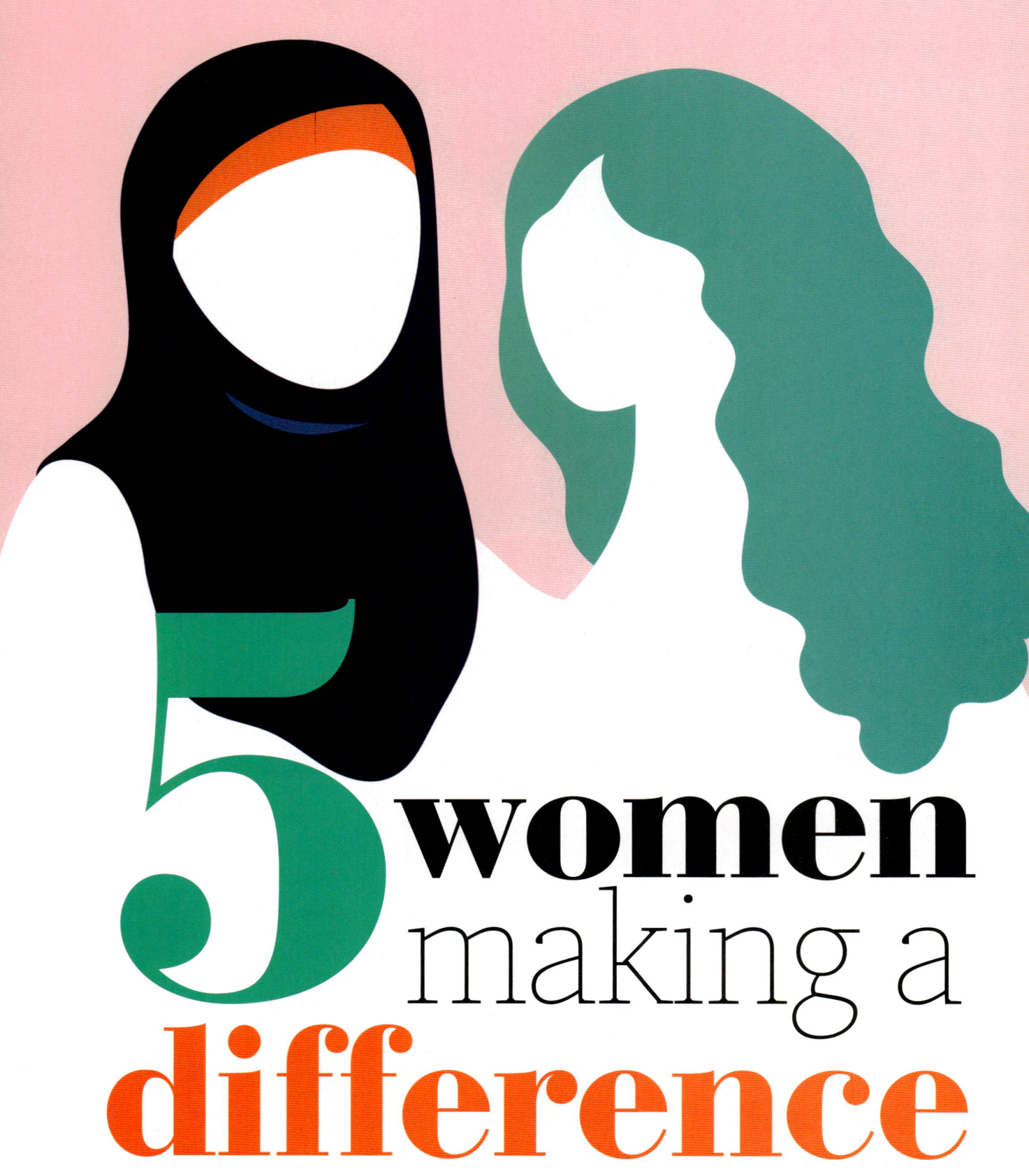

5 women making a difference

Menopause is no longer hiding in the shadows, and the right support is on the rise, thanks to women like these…

EXPERIENCE

'The medical world needs to be more tuned in'

THE DOCTOR

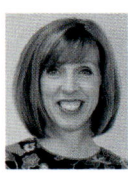

Dr Louise Newson is a GP specialising in perimenopause and menopause. Her work focuses on women having access to the right treatment and also challenging misinformation around HRT. In 2018, she opened the dedicated menopause clinic Newson Health Menopause and Wellbeing Centre (newsonhealth.co.uk), and she runs a website (menopausedoctor.co.uk) to provide evidence-based advice.

'We did a survey of 3,000 menopausal women, and 66% of them had been given antidepressants when they went to see their GP about perimenopausal or menopausal symptoms. Others have been incorrectly told that it's just a natural process to ride out, that HRT is too risky or that they're too young to start HRT. The reality is that HRT can transform women who are suffering from debilitating symptoms, such as brain fog, mood swings and severe anxiety, and give them their lives back. It also helps reduce your risk of heart disease and osteoporosis.

'The way that it should be prescribed is through patient choice. This means fully educating the patient of the risks vs benefits and making a decision based on that – not just denying them a chance to have it.

'I run courses training doctors and nurses about the menopause and HRT – all medical disciplines need to be more tuned into menopause, from psychiatry to urology, because many symptoms women are experiencing that are related to the menopause – such as anxiety, fatigue, worsening migraines and repeated urinary tract infections – are too often missed.'

'I realised something needed to be done in the workplace'

THE CAMPAIGNER

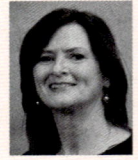

Karen Wright, 52, is the Assistant Director of Workforce for Velindre University NHS Trust in Wales. Karen initiated huge menopause support in her Trust, and her ideas are spreading to other organisations.

'In 2014, I had chemo for breast cancer. When I went back to work months later, I still felt awful – I had extreme fatigue, hot flushes, brain fog, poor memory and my confidence was on the floor. I went back to my consultant and he told me that the chemo had put me into early menopause.

'I was on the verge of resigning because I wasn't coping, but, after talking with a trade-union officer about the TUC's 'menopause toolkit', I knew something needed to be done to provide menopause support in the workplace.

'Our executive board was supportive, so I set up the first Workplace Menopause Café in Wales. It was a great success and we now have several events each year, plus clinics where medical professionals come to advise staff.

'I've introduced menopause buddies – people who volunteer to support their colleagues – plus clear guidelines for managers, including a menopause question on return-to-work forms. Our Trust workforce is 75% female, and 64% of those are 40-60+, so it makes sense to provide the support to retain them!'

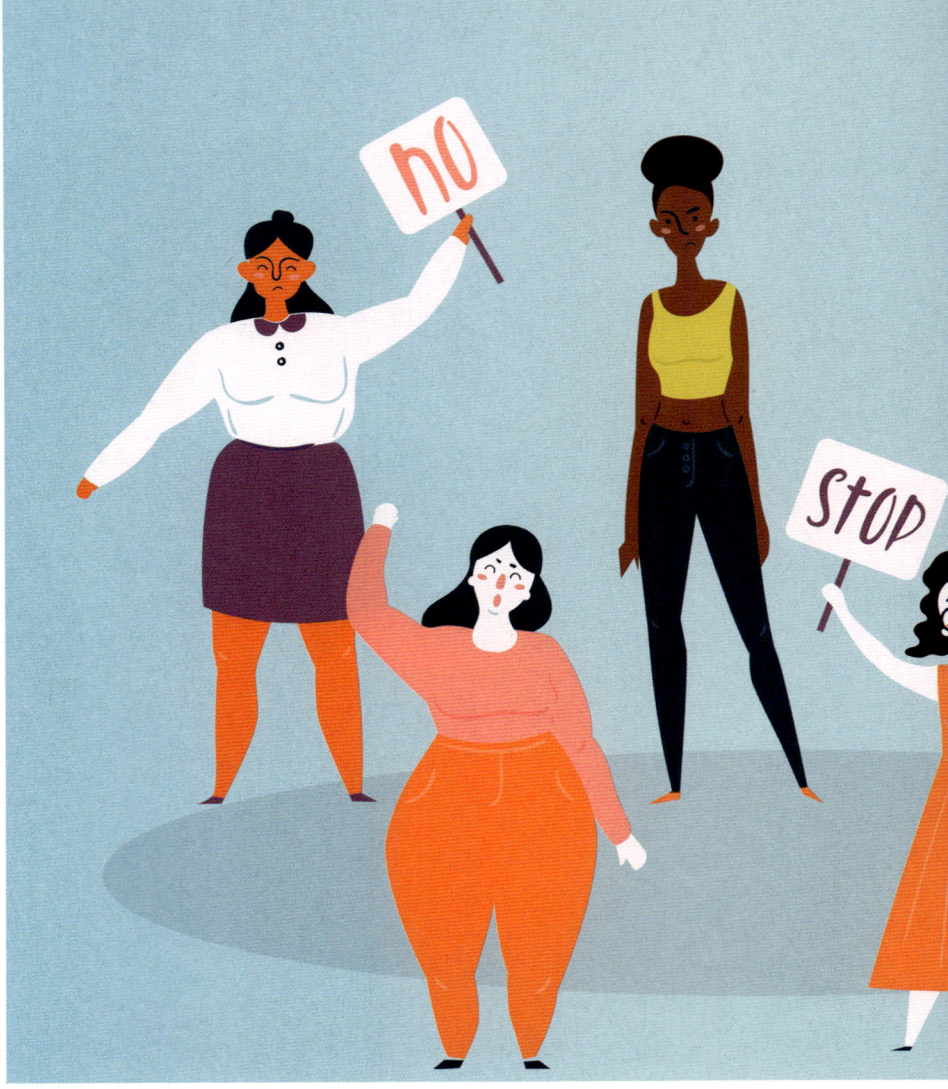

THE PSYCHOTHERAPIST

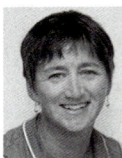

Diane Danzebrink is a psychotherapist with a special interest in menopause. She counsels women and couples through menopause, but also became a campaigner after a shockingly awful experience of surgically-induced menopause at 45.

She is founder of the #MakeMenopause Matter campaign (menopausesupport.co.uk), which aims to improve menopause education amongst GPs, raise awareness within the workplace and introduce menopause education into the curriculum for teenage boys and girls.

'The silver lining to my terrible experience of menopause is everything that's happened since. Our campaign now has cross-party political support and teaching about the menopause for both sexes is going to be included in the school curriculum from September 2020.

'It's vital that men know about menopause, too, as they will work with, live with or be friends with women. My motto is that if you are a woman, know a woman or love a woman, you need to know about menopause!'

'When I was at my lowest, I rang my GP surgery and asked if there were any menopause support groups and was told, "No, I'm sorry, dear, there's nothing like that". That feeling of being alone with it almost broke me and I vowed that, once I was better, I would change things for other women.'

> 'If you are a woman, know a woman or love a woman, you need to know'

EXPERIENCE

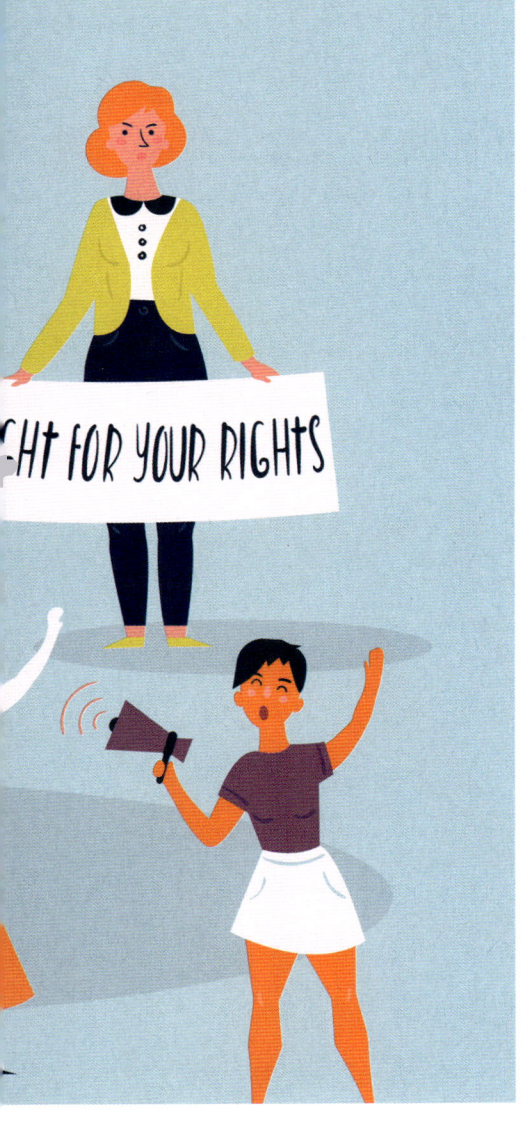

THE THEATRE DIRECTOR

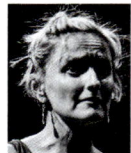

Claire Hodgson, 48, is a theatre, dance and circus director (diversecity.org.uk). She has created a play called *Mid Life,* which explores menopause and the life stories of middle-aged women. It was performed at the Barbican in February 2020 and at the Bristol Old Vic in March 2020 (barbican.org.uk; bristololdvic.org.uk).

'When I was 44, I started to feel very anxious and exhausted. It wasn't until my partner suggested that it could be to do with menopause (he's older and has female friends who've been through it) that I had any idea what was happening.

'As a director, my instinct was to create a show about it to bring menopause into the arts space in a performance that I would have wanted to see to help me feel less alone. So, with two theatre colleagues and a writer, we began sessions of storytelling about our lives and menopause, to start building the show.

'We also interviewed our mums and women from all kinds of backgrounds – menopause is too often portrayed as silver-haired, white women wearing linen and walking on a beach, and I wanted the show to be more representative of all women of all ages. We're having children later, so some of us are already menopausal at the school gates!

'I am in the show, as are my two co-creators, although two of us aren't usually actors. The play is about reflecting on your past, grief and loss, but also about the positives of becoming yourself and removing the shame about getting older.'

> 'We celebrate the positives of becoming yourself'

THE CAFÉ FOUNDER

Rachel Weiss, 53, is a counsellor, coach and founder of the hugely successful Menopause Café movement (menopausecafe.net), where people

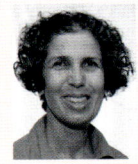

gather in cafés across the UK and other countries to 'eat cake, drink tea and discuss menopause'.

She also created FlushFest, an annual festival designed to break taboos, with comedians, cabaret and creative workshops alongside talks from menopause specialists.

'I was inspired to set up Menopause Café (based on the existing Death Café model) after watching Kirsty Wark's *The Menopause and Me* in 2017. I hadn't experienced menopause, but I could see that there was a need for a space for people to come together and talk about what was happening to them or their loved ones.

'With two other women, I held the first-ever meeting in a café in Perth, Scotland. Word spread, Kirsty Wark became our patron and, by January 2018, we had our first cafés outside Scotland; in March 2018, we had our first outside the UK – in Toronto. Now there are hundreds of events each year.

'Participants sit in small groups to share stories, offer support and exchange tips. People often say they get a feeling of relief to that they're not alone and they're not going mad.'

> 'Women are relieved to feel they are not alone'

There's more help out there...

Find more amazing women and feel supported:
On Twitter:
- **@menopause_talk** – Ruth Devlin, author of *Men...Let's Talk Menopause*
- **@henpickednet** – Deborah Garlick and her brilliant content for 'women who weren't born yesterday'
- **@pausitivity2** – the successful #knowyourmenopause poster campaign

Online:
- **Women's Health Concern (WHC) is the patient arm of the British Menopause Society (BMS),** providing a confidential, independent service to women of all ages. There's plenty of support material on both websites: womens-health-concern.org; thebms.org.uk

The smart guide menopause QUIZ

Been paying attention? Test your knowledge and keep your symptoms in check

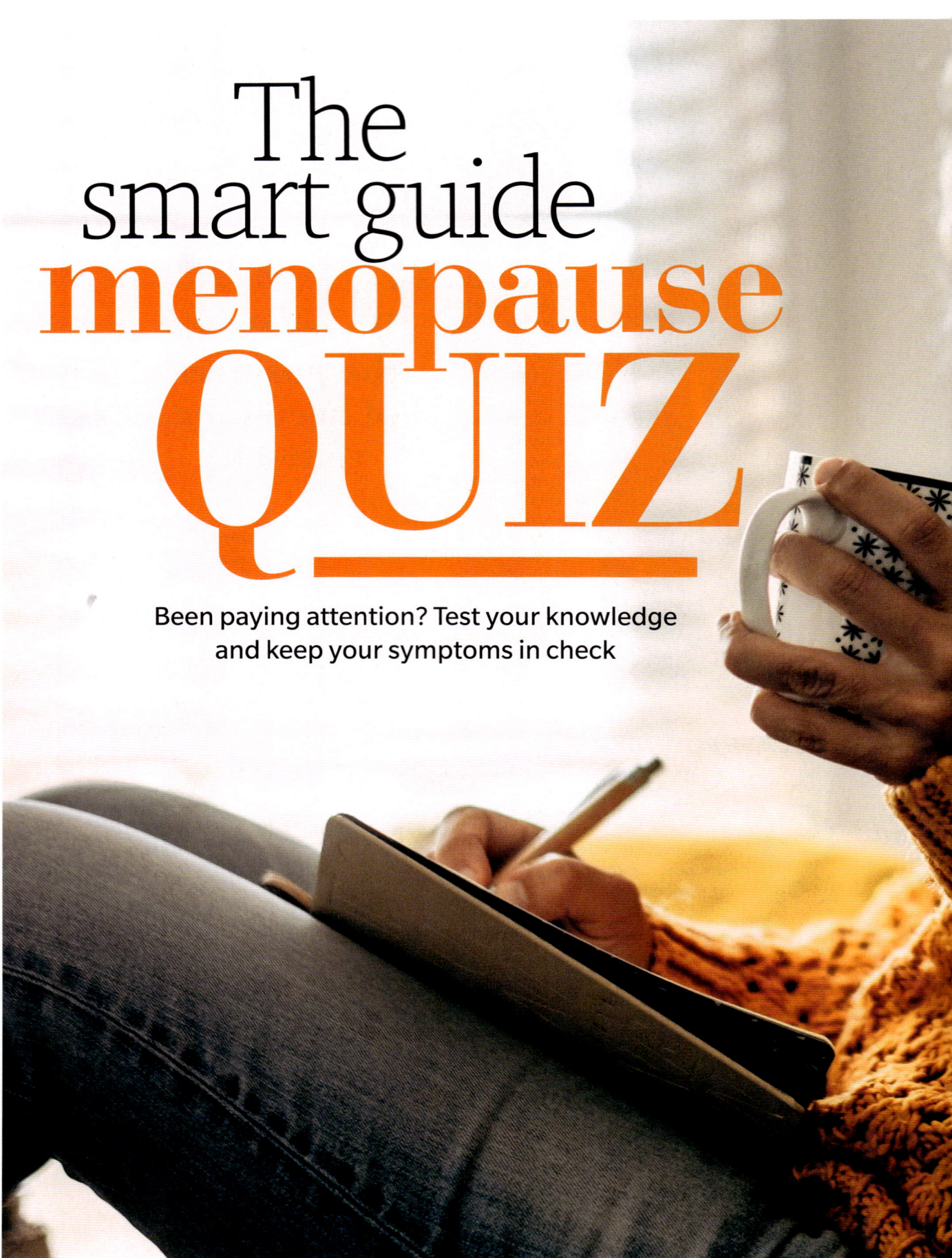

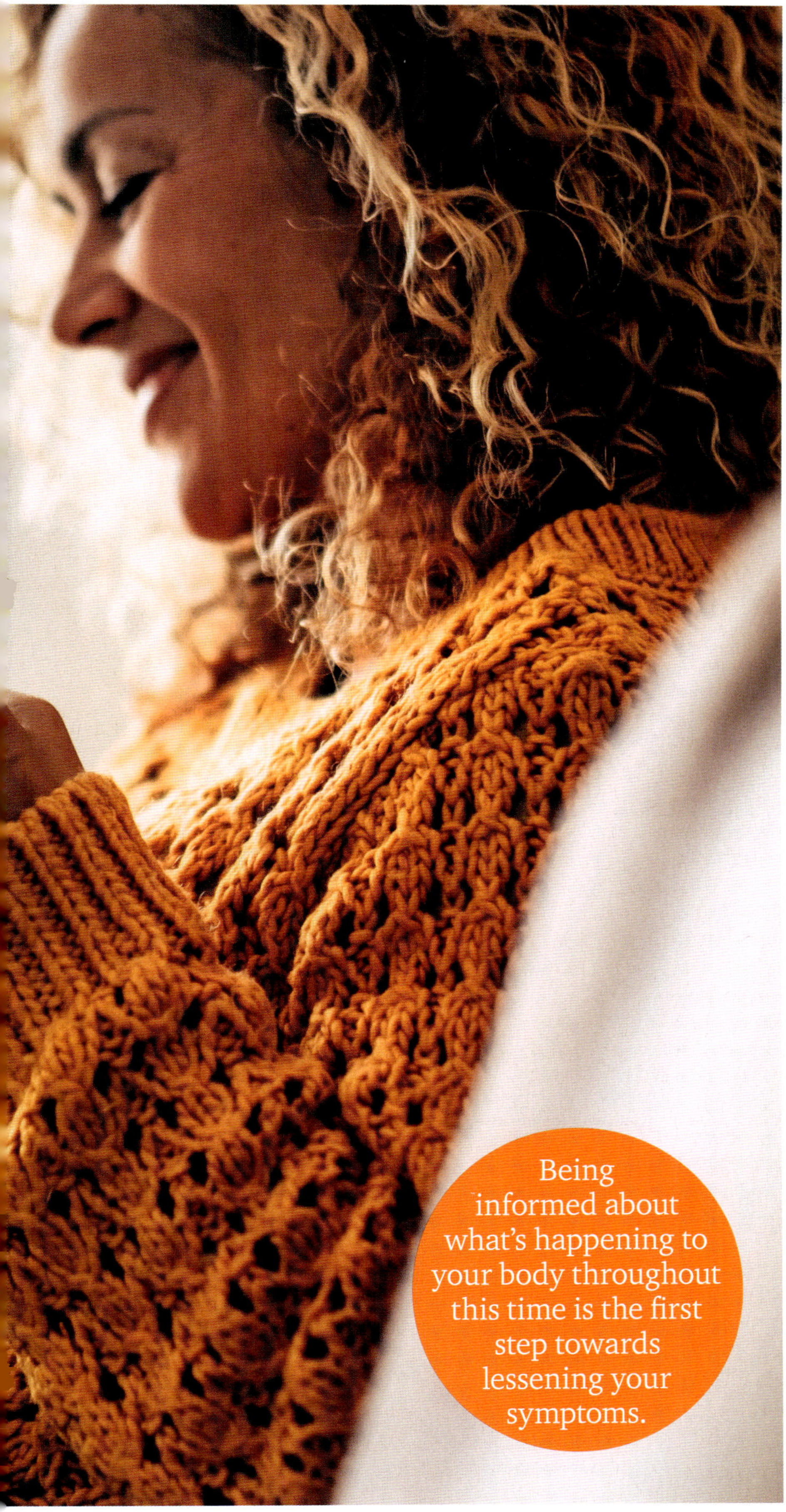

WHAT DO YOU KNOW?

1 Which foods are better to avoid?
A Spicy
B Soya
ANSWER: Spicy. They're a notorious stimulant and likely to trigger night sweats and hot flushes if you're one of the 85% of menopausal women who get them. By contrast a US study of over 1,200 women found that two portions of soya foods daily could reduce hot flushes by 26%.

2 Which habit should you kick first?
A Cigarettes
B Alcohol
ANSWER: Cigarettes. Smoking speeds up oestrogen loss, bringing on menopause symptoms earlier, according to a study from Pennsylvania. But that doesn't mean alcohol isn't to be avoided or at least reduced – it can increase your risk of hot flushes in the same way as spicy foods do, so limiting your intake is a good idea. It also speeds up the bone changes that can lead to osteoporosis.

3 Which is the better alcoholic drink option?
A White wine
B Red wine
ANSWER: White wine. While all alcohol can cause an epinephrine release, which can trigger a hot flush, red wine is particularly potent. But, as with any alcoholic drink, it's always best to remember safe drinking guidelines and indulge in moderation to stay healthy.

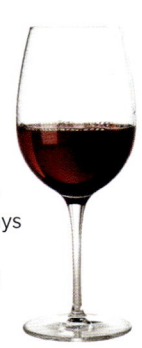

4 Which is the lesser of two evils?
A Salt
B Sugar
ANSWER: Both are as bad as each other. Sugar encourages hot flushes, but the hormonal changes during menopause can make you more sensitive to salt, which can lead to raised blood pressure – a major risk factor for stroke and heart disease.

> Being informed about what's happening to your body throughout this time is the first step towards lessening your symptoms.

The Smart Woman's Guide to the Menopause

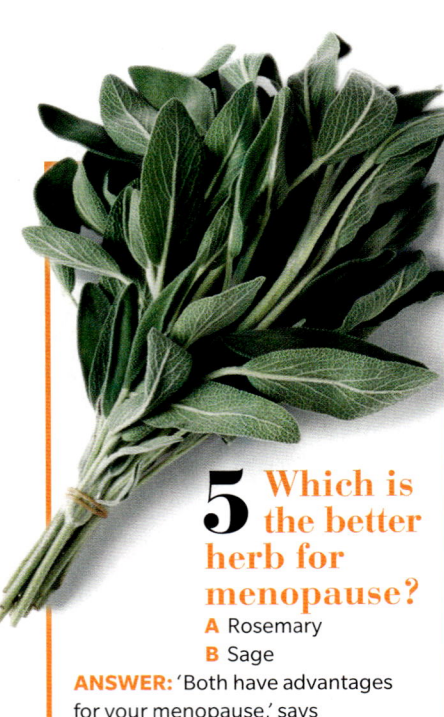

5 Which is the better herb for menopause?
A Rosemary
B Sage
ANSWER: 'Both have advantages for your menopause,' says nutritionist Judy Watson (judywatsonnutritionist.co.uk). Choose sage to prevent hot flushes and rosemary as a memory booster.

6 When should you give up using contraception?
A One year after your periods stop
B Two years after your periods stop
ANSWER: 'One year after the age of 50, but two years if you're younger,' says Dr Heather Currie, gynaecologist and Managing Director of menopause matters.co.uk.

7 Which is safer to take in menopause?
A Bioidentical hormones
B HRT
ANSWER: HRT. 'Most HRT formulations are plant-based and "bioidentical" (meaning they're an exact match for what your body would naturally make), but the point is that only prescribed HRTs are guaranteed to be made to rigorous safety standards,' says Dr Currie.

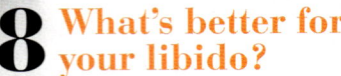

8 What's better for your libido?
A Testosterone
B Oestrogen
ANSWER: 'The oestrogen in most HRT formulations should help, but when it's not doing the trick your doctor can prescribe another formula with added testosterone for an extra boost,' says Dr Currie. 'But there are many other factors also affecting a woman's libido that hormones cannot help – you may need some psychosexual therapy, for example.'

9 Progestogen should always be used alongside oestrogen…
A True?
B False?
ANSWER: False. 'Progestogen is needed to prevent womb cancer, which becomes a risk if you take oestrogen alone. But women who have had a hysterectomy have no need for this. And you do not need it if you use a local (vaginal) oestrogen, although some GPs are confused about this,' says Dr Currie.

10 Which are the better fats to include?
A Omega-3s
B Saturated fats
ANSWER: Omega-3 fats. 'These lubricate the body and can help with a number of symptoms we associate with menopause, including dry hair, skin and nails, and even vaginal dryness,' says women's health specialist Dr Marilyn Glenville, author of *Natural Solutions To Menopause* (£12.99, Rodale).

11 For painful sex you'd use:
A A vaginal moisturiser?
B An oestrogen cream?
ANSWER: Either or both. Painful sex is a symptom for 84% of women after menopause. 'A vaginal moisturiser can help but if it's not enough your GP can prescribe a vaginal cream, vaginal tablets or a vaginal ring containing oestrogen to increase the flow of natural lubrication,' says Dr Currie.

12 Which are better for your waistline?
A Carbohydrates
B Proteins
ANSWER: Proteins. 'Your hormonal shifts make you more insulin-sensitive around menopause, encouraging more fat storage from diets high in carbs,' says Judy. 'You're also losing muscle mass after 40, making it harder to burn off calories.'

13 The best exercise for you now is:
A A mindful stroll
B A power walk
ANSWER: A power walk. You'll release mood-enhancing endorphins while also keeping menopausal weight gain at bay, lowering your risk of breast cancer and strengthening your bones against osteoporosis.

Unsure of anything? Why not read the relevant pages again?

14 In order to improve your bladder control, which should you do:
A Pelvic floor contractions
B Sit-ups
ANSWER: At least 100 contractions daily will strengthen your pelvic-floor muscles. Conversely, sit-ups can put pressure on a weak pelvic floor and lead to a prolapsed bladder or uterus.

15 Which yogurt is better for you?
A Plain
B Fruit
ANSWER: Plain – and full-fat Greek, for preference, says Judy. 'It's an excellent source of calcium, which you need for bone health. The average 150g fruit yogurt contains six teaspoons of sugar.'

WHAT DO YOU KNOW?

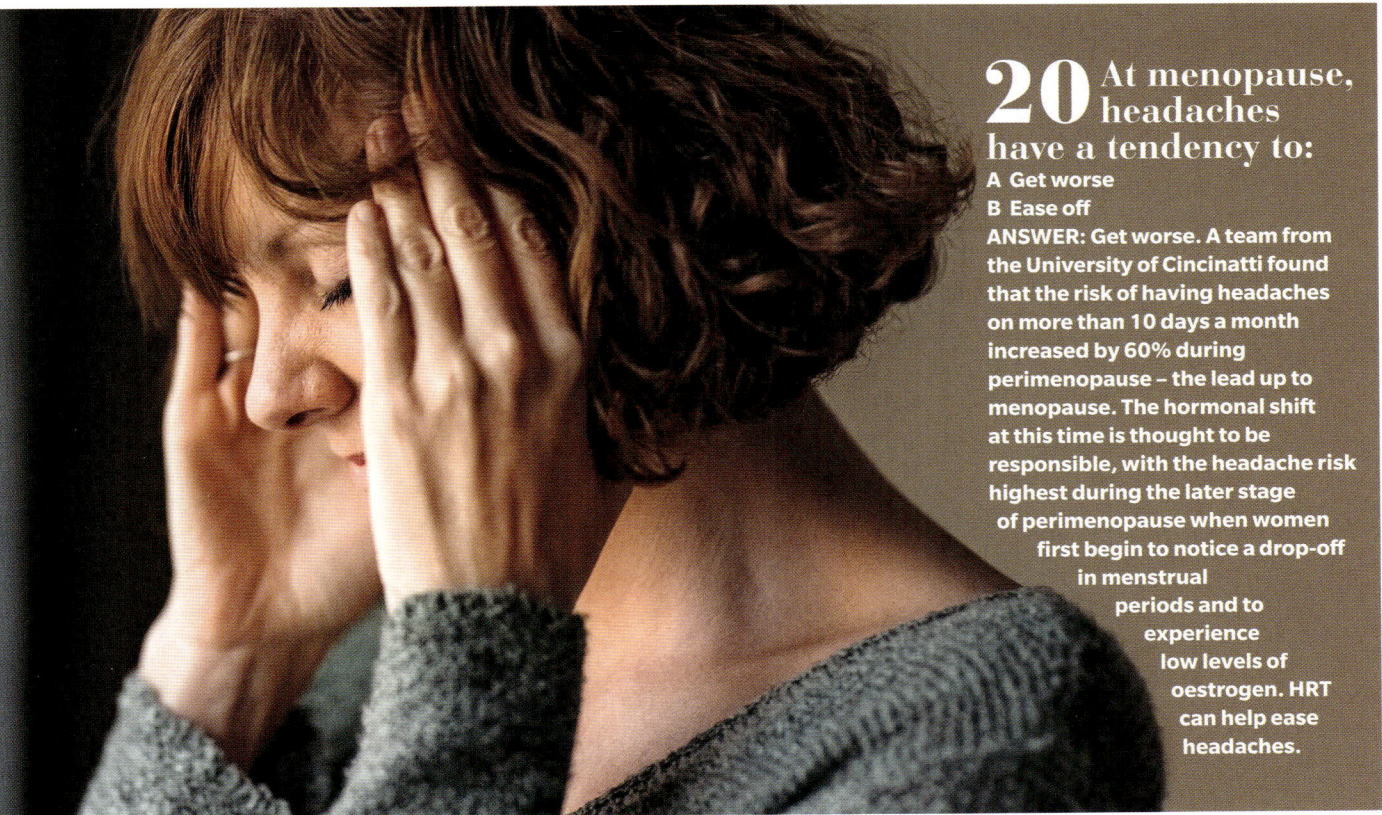

20 At menopause, headaches have a tendency to:
A Get worse
B Ease off
ANSWER: Get worse. A team from the University of Cincinatti found that the risk of having headaches on more than 10 days a month increased by 60% during perimenopause – the lead up to menopause. The hormonal shift at this time is thought to be responsible, with the headache risk highest during the later stage of perimenopause when women first begin to notice a drop-off in menstrual periods and to experience low levels of oestrogen. HRT can help ease headaches.

16 Probiotics are:
A Useful at menopause
B Irrelevant
ANSWER: Useful. 'These healthy bugs reduce your risk of weight gain, and they also support your liver in helping with the breakdown of oestrogens in your body,' says Judy.

17 Which hot drink is most beneficial in menopause?
A Hot chocolate
B Green tea
ANSWER: Green tea. 'It's low in caffeine (a stimulant for hot flushes) and helps with circulation, as heart problems are an increased risk,' says Judy.

18 Which seeds help most with night sweats?
A Flaxseeds
B Pumpkin seeds
ANSWER: Flaxseeds. A six-week Mayo Clinic study gave 29 women 40g of ground flaxseed daily and saw the frequency of their flushing drop by 50% and the severity by 57%. They reported better moods and less joint/muscle pain, too.

19 Menopausal memory loss is:
A A myth
B Something you'll get over eventually
ANSWER: Something you'll get over – usually after about a year. US researchers found that the worse a woman's hot flushes, the worse her memory loss will be in menopause, too.

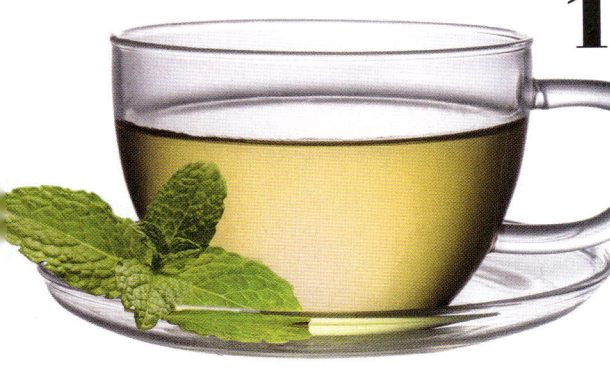

HOW DID YOU DO?

16-20 CORRECT ANSWERS
Congratulations! You're quite a menopause mastermind – now make sure you're putting all that great knowledge into practice.

6-15 CORRECT ANSWERS
Great effort! We've hopefully shone some light on a few new areas for you to brush up on, but your menopause knowledge is pretty good!

5 CORRECT ANSWERS OR LESS
Time to revisit some of the information contained in this magazine. Our expert tips and information really can help you through this time in your life, so don't miss out.

The Smart Woman's Guide to the Menopause

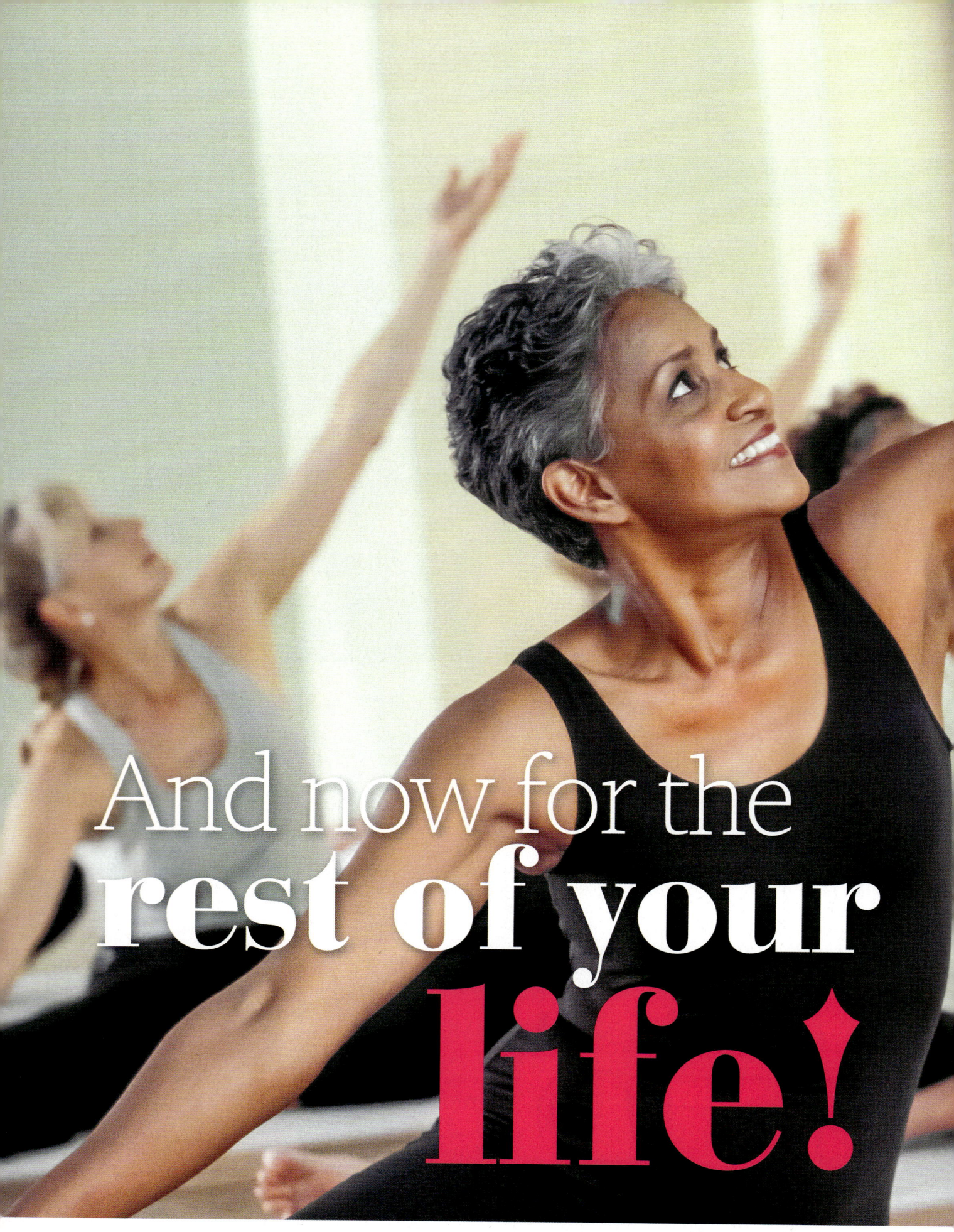

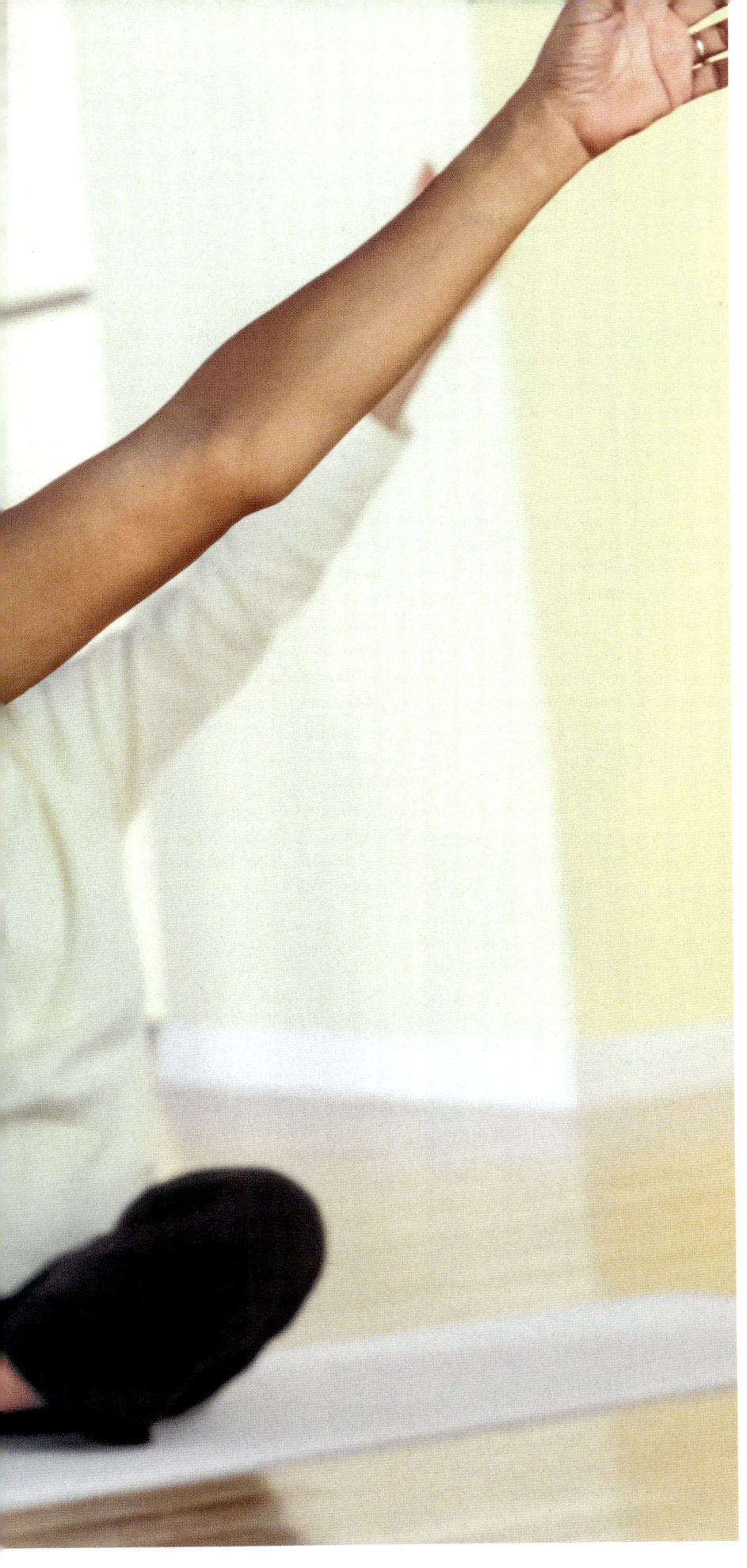

SELF-ESTEEM

You're through the menopause and out the other side. Now it's time to restore that oomph by rebuilding your confidence. Here's good advice from the experts…

You might be wondering what on earth happened to the person you were before menopause. It could be you've emerged feeling less the life and soul and more the invisible woman.

A confidence report from Dove Beauty found that nine out of 10 women opt out of important life activities when they don't feel good about how they look. It also found that the same amount of us have put our health at risk by messing about with diets, due to lack of self-esteem. These shocking statistics shed light on the ever-growing issue of poor self-belief and overwhelming insecurity among Brits – particularly women who have been through the menopause. Sound familiar? Here's how to overcome your own confidence crisis.

Look ahead…

Celebrate the menopause (yes really!). In traditional Chinese medicine, a woman's menopause is called 'second spring', and celebrated as the gateway to an energetic and independent older age that women can look forward to. You are now rid of your periods and can also say goodbye to PMS and menstrual migraines.

'Some women find their libido surges after menopause, and of course, you no longer have to worry about contraception,' says menopause expert Dr Heather Currie (menopausematters.co.uk). 'If you've suffered with fibroids – which affect one in three women – these tend to stop growing, or even shrink, once you've had your menopause and oestrogen levels drop.'

The Smart Woman's Guide to the Menopause

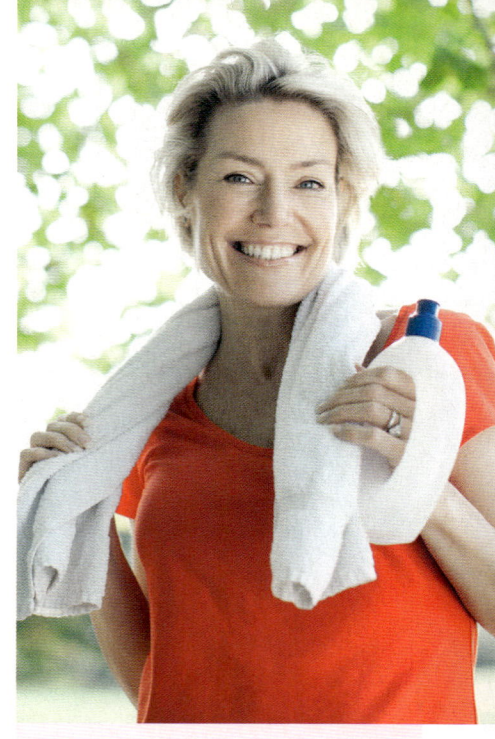

Focus on your FRIENDS AND FAMILY

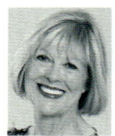

Psychotherapist Christine Webber is the author of *Get The Self-Esteem Habit* (available at amazon.co.uk).

Rethink your relationship with your grown children. The transition from dependent child to fully fledged adult can be tricky and you want your relationship to be strong and intact at the end of it. Remember, they can no longer be expected to do what you tell them. Seeing them outside the domestic context – at the theatre, out for a meal, a shopping trip – can help.

Nurture other family relationships. Research shows that as we get older and think more about our past, our relationship with siblings becomes more important to our happiness. They're the people who knew you best before life got complicated. Create a family group text, WhatsApp or Facebook page. Arrange get-togethers and if there are other family members, such as cousins, include them too.

Learn from your children. You've seen how vital friends are to your children – but the demands of family, home and career means we have often neglected ours. Set up a regular slot with a colleague or neighbour – aerobics on Wednesday evenings, lunch Fridays?

Follow your passions. See this new space as a chance to put yourself centre stage. Are there residential courses or night classes that inspire you? Whether it's guerrilla gardening or volunteering at a stately home, following your passions will open new doors and introduce like-minded people.

Focus on your HEALTH

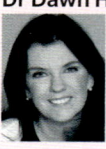

Dr Dawn Harper is the author of *Live Well to 101* (£9.99, Headline Home).

Concentrate on small, achievable changes. Think of this as a pension policy – the more you pay in, the more you stand to gain.

Get physical. The NHS aim is 150 minutes per week of moderate exercise or 75 minutes of vigorous exercise, though you can start with modest targets: 'I'll walk to work on Thursdays' or 'I won't sit when I could stand'.

Tackle bad habits. Smokers are four times more likely to quit if they do it with help – free with the NHS. When drinking, try having a couple of dry days a week.

Give your brain a workout. When you learn something new and difficult, you grow new neural connections and strengthen weak ones. Set small mental challenges – wean off the calculator or memorise a poem – or launch big ones, such as learning a language.

Don't miss health checks. If you haven't had one for a while, contact your GP to see if you are eligible. Find out as much as possible about your family health history – and if it suggests inherited risk of cancers or heart disease, ask about screening.

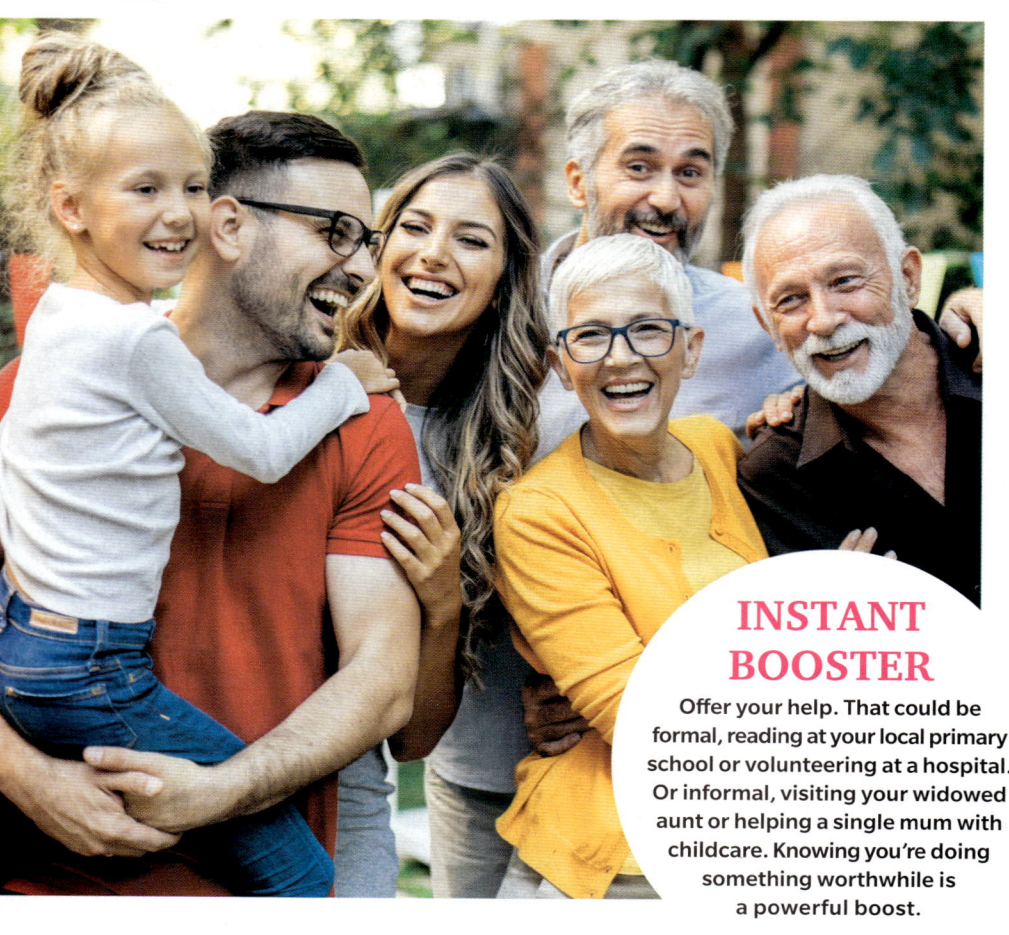

INSTANT BOOSTER

Offer your help. That could be formal, reading at your local primary school or volunteering at a hospital. Or informal, visiting your widowed aunt or helping a single mum with childcare. Knowing you're doing something worthwhile is a powerful boost.

SELF-ESTEEM

INSTANT BOOSTER

Value your age. Younger women are quick to act, but they can make mistakes because they haven't thought things through. Older women, on the other hand, know what doesn't work. They may be slower because they're considering all the options but they can be more effective.

INSTANT BOOSTER

Promise yourself the gift of me time from now on – whether that's an extra hour in bed, a blank day in the diary, lunch with a friend or a long walk. Committing to putting yourself high on the agenda is important for you and everyone else. When you've made that leap, you're halfway there.

Focus on your CAREER

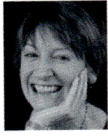

Sue Clarke is a career coach (inthehotseat.co.uk)
Examine and identify the career changes you want to see. Is it that you're not developing, or can't get organised, or you feel overlooked?

Choose one area, then devise a plan. If you try changing everything at once, it's overwhelming. A career coach is helpful here. If you want to make a big change, even switch careers, look at all the possibilities. Can you downsize to free up financial responsibilities? Can you return to higher education?

Find your tribe. Create a list of 'older women champions' through work, LinkedIn and professional networks who are doing what you'd like to do, and women who have moved up or changed roles in the way you'd like to.

Don't wait to be noticed. Feeling invisible at work is common in midlife. Don't wait to be invited to meetings or conferences, don't wait to be asked to contribute. If you feel sidelined, overlooked for opportunities, put your name forward. If you're not informed about a meeting and feel it's relevant, go and explain why you're there.

Put yourself forward as a mentor. Making a positive contribution boosts confidence and mentoring will prove to you – and everyone else – the value of wisdom and experience.

The Smart Woman's Guide to the Menopause

Be free, be brave, be HAPPY!

Wave goodbye to taboos and celebrate your new-found liberty says psychologist and author Dr Megan A. Arroll. Good times are on their way!

When a cloud of taboo surrounds a topic, we miss out on important opportunities to communicate our feelings and experiences. And if there's a sense of shame, stigma or embarrassment about our symptoms, we're less likely to open up about what we're going through – which can increase the likelihood of anxiety, depression and a sense of isolation. In menopause, this means missing out on the support, good quality medical advice and care that is needed to navigate an often confusing and bewildering maze of symptoms.

The experience of menopause has been hidden behind closed doors for far too long, and now it's time to say goodbye to this antiquated taboo. Over the past few years, we've seen women smash unhelpful stereotypes of 'the menopausal woman' with mainstream campaigns and documentaries, a powerful voice on social media and notable figures sharing their experiences.

This goes a long way – and we must also highlight the wealth of research showing the benefits of midlife, including a boost in confidence, feeling free and liberated from the concerns of menstruation and pregnancy, and an increased sense of attractiveness. A recent poll of 2,000 women aged 50 and above, commissioned by leading supplement provider Healthspan, found 72% of women feel their overall confidence depends on how they feel about their appearance.

Midlife is a wonderful time to take risks in life. What were all those things you wanted to do but didn't have time, were too preoccupied with the kids or simply didn't feel brave enough? We're living for longer, but the average age of menopause hasn't changed, so it's possible that you still have half your life

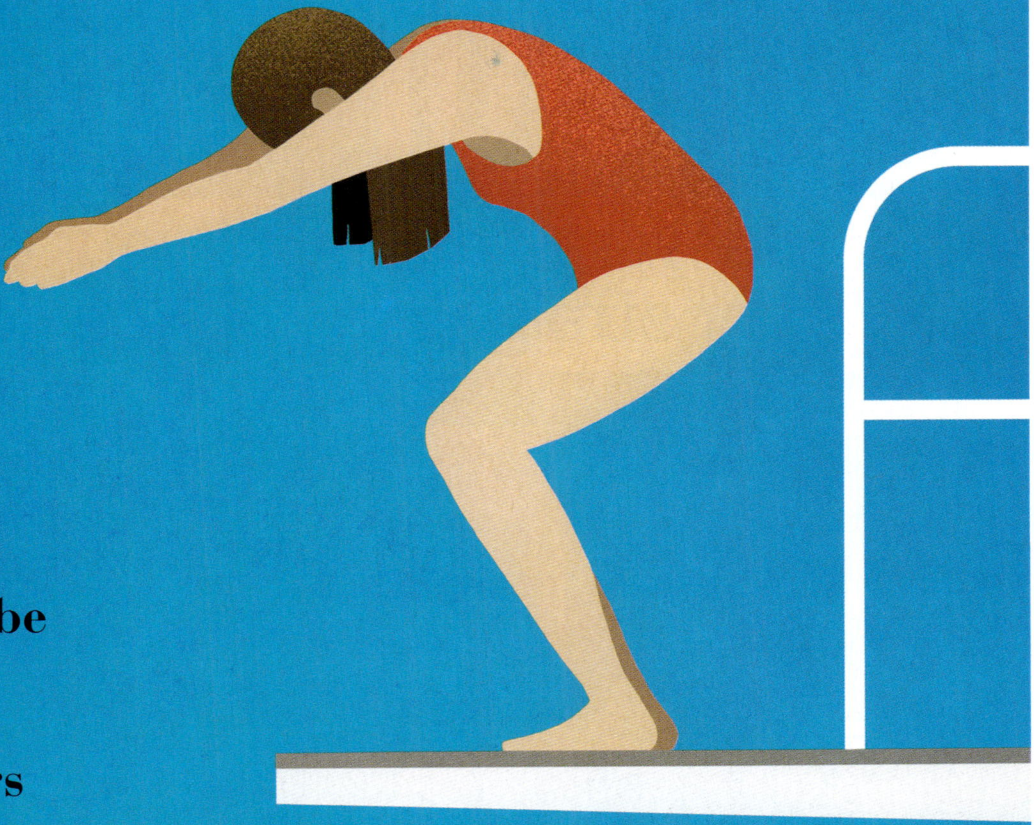

LAST WORD

> **It's possible for these to be some of the most active, healthy years of your life**

to live – so go out there and truly live it!

With good self-care, it's possible for these to be some of the most active and healthy years of your life. Many women now get fit in their 40s and 50s, learn new skills, travel and more frequently change careers. With the experience and knowledge you'll have acquired, kids – if you had them – no longer in the nest and fewer concerns over what others think, it's all now enormously possible.

This is your time – a chance to live out your dreams. Focus on you, look after yourself and be fearless!

Chartered psychologist Dr Megan A. Arroll is co-author of The Menopause Maze: The Complete Guide to Conventional, Complementary and Self-Help Options (£12.99, Singing Dragon).

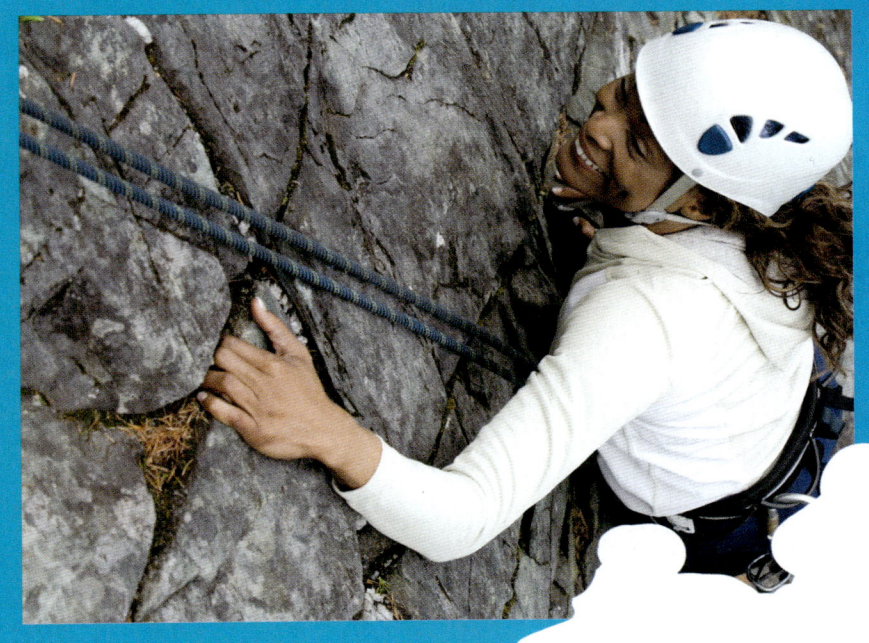

SUBSCRIBE & SAVE UP TO 61%

Delivered direct to your door or straight to your device

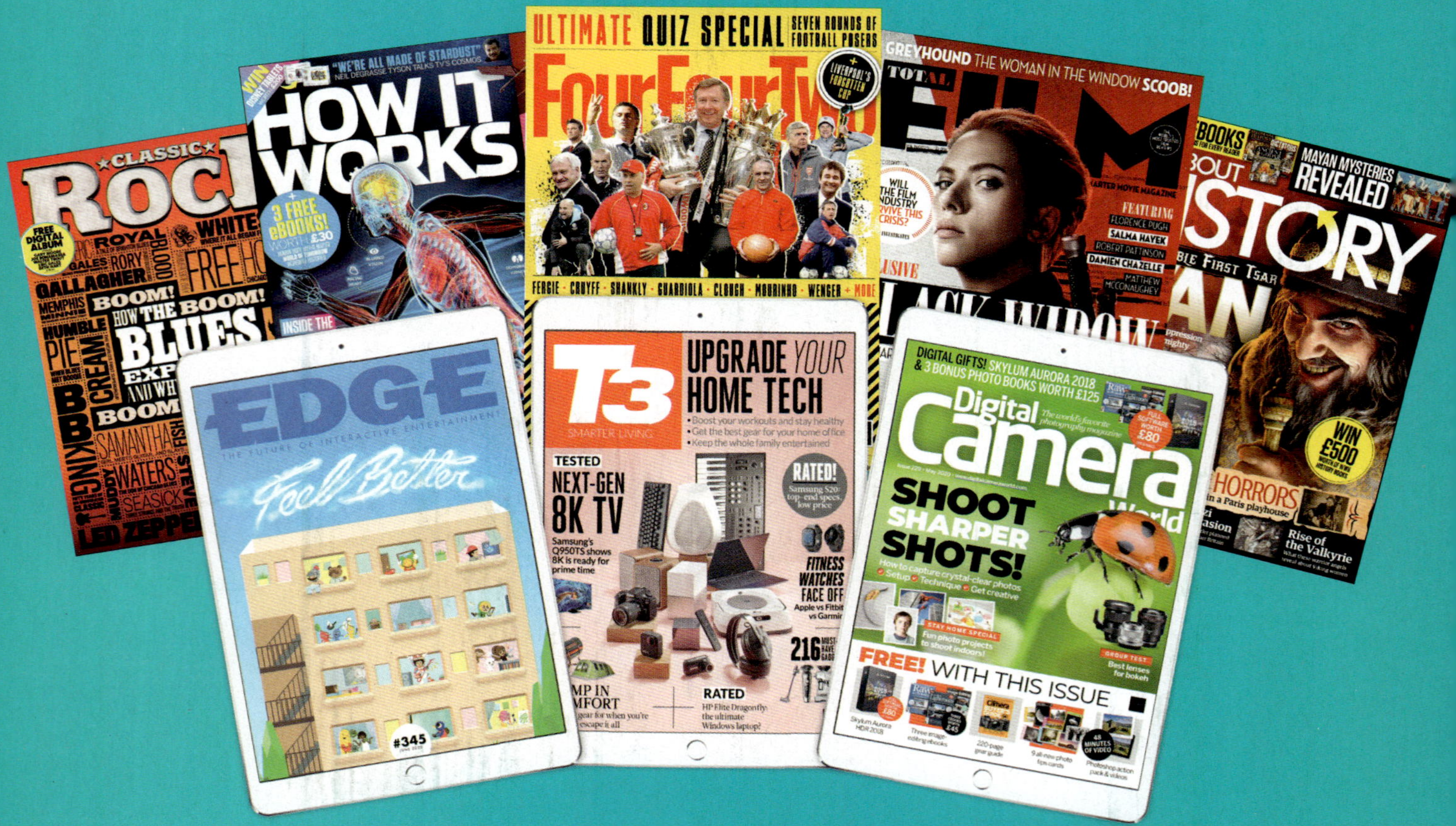

Choose from over 80 magazines and make great savings off the store price!

Binders, books and back issues also available

Simply visit www.magazinesdirect.com

✓ No hidden costs 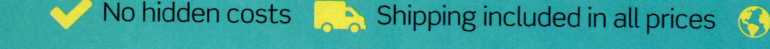 Shipping included in all prices 🌐 We deliver to over 100 countries 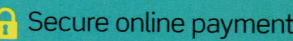 Secure online payment

FUTURE

magazinesdirect.com
Official Magazine Subscription Store